T0250493

Moving with the Times

Moving with the Times

*Gender, Status and Migration
of Nurses in India*

SREELEKHA NAIR

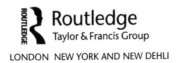

LONDON NEW YORK AND NEW DEHLI

First published 2012 in India
by Routledge
912 Tolstoy House, 15–17 Tolstoy Marg, Connaught Place, New Delhi 110 001

Simultaneously published in the UK
by Routledge
2 Park Square, Milton Park, Abingdon, Oxfordshire OX14 4RN

First issued in paperback 2015

Routledge is an imprint of the Taylor & Francis Group, an informa business

Typeset by
Star Compugraphics Private Limited
5, CSC, Near City Apartments
Vasundhara Enclave
Delhi 110 096

British Library Cataloguing-in-Publication Data
A catalogue record of this book is available from the British Library

ISBN 13: 978-1-138-66258-2 (pbk)
ISBN 13: 978-0-415-54061-2 (hbk)

Contents

List of Tables and Figures

Tables

Figures

List of Abbreviations

AIIMS	All India Institute of Medical Sciences
ANM	Auxiliary Nurse-Midwife
ANS	Association of Nursing Superintendents
CGFNS	Commission on Graduates of Foreign Nursing Schools
CPI (M)	Communist Party of India (Marxist)
CV	Curriculum Vitae
CWDS	Centre for Women's Development Studies
DNU	Delhi Nurses' Union
KEM Hospital	King Edward Memorial Hospital
GNM	General Nursing and Midwifery
HIV/AIDS	Human Immunodeficiency Virus/Acquired Immunodeficiency Syndrome
ICN	International Council of Nurses
ICU	Intensive Care Unit
IELTS	International English Language Testing System
INC	Indian Nursing Council
JMS	Janwadi Mahila Samiti
MNWA	Malayali Nurses' Welfare Association
NFIW	National Federation of Indian Women
NHS	National Health Service
NRSI	Nursing Research Society of India
TNA	Trained Nurses' Association
TNAI	Trained Nurses' Association of India
US	United States
UK	United Kingdom
UNICEF	United Nations Children's Fund
USAID	United States Agency for International Development

Glossary

asura	A negative supernatural being in Hinduism
avatar	Incarnation or manifestation of a supreme deity in Hinduism
ayah	maid, servant or nursemaid
Ayyappa	A deity worshipped mainly in south India, believed to be born out of the union between Vishnu and Shiva.
bahar	outside the home/public spaces
Brahminical	The system that perpetuates the cultural, social and economic practices of Brahmins, the traditional elite or priestly caste in Hindu society.
Chamar	A former untouchable caste found in the northern states of India whose main occupation was processing, manufacturing and trading in leather and leather goods
Charaka	Referred to sometimes as the father of the ancient Indian system of medicine and lifestyle, Ayurveda.
dai	Traditional midwife in some parts of South Asia
Dalit	Term used by former untouchable caste groups in South Asia for themselves
dawai	Medicine
denewali	giver, provider
deva	Benevolent supernatural being or God, opposite of asura.
dil	Heart
dosa	An equivalent of crepes or pancakes made from the fermented batter of rice and black lentils. A staple dish of southern India and Sri Lanka.
Ezhava	A former backward caste in Kerala, known also as Chokon and Thiyya who were mainly

	agricultural labourers, small cultivators and toddy-tappers.
ghar	Home/domestic space
Hindi	Official language of the northern states of India; also used as the official language of the Republic of India along with English
idli	Steamed, salted cake made from the fermented batter of rice and black lentils. The staple breakfast dish of the southern states of India.
Indra	The king of the devas and the lord of the heavens.
infirmière	Nurse (in French)
Kaliyugam	The last of the four stages of the cycle of time that the world goes through. It is condemned for its moral decay according to the Hindu scriptures.
Kudumba mahima	Family reputation and honour
Madrasi	Term used in ignorant typecasting of people from south India as hailing from Madras, with a derogatory connotation.
Mahabali	Benevolent asura king of the present region of Kerala associated with the Onam festival
mala	Hill
Malayali	A person whose mother tongue is Malayalam, originally from Kerala
mangalsutr	A gold chain with beads worn by married women in many communities in north India; its equivalent in south India is a pendant called *Thali*.
Marumakkathayam	A system of inheritance, descent and succession to property through female members of the family which prevailed in the past among communities like Nairs in Kerala.
methrani	Helper
Onam	Harvest festival of Kerala celebrating the homecoming of the legendary emperor Mahabali.

pardeshi	Foreigner/person who has no entitlement to a place
pathala	The world under earth where Mahabali was sent by Vamana, Vishnu's incarnation
Perunnal	Local festival and feast of Christian churches in Kerala
pettachi	Midwife in Kerala
pooja or puja	Religious ritual and worship
pothujanam	General public
pravasi	Non-resident
Punjabi	Language of Punjab or the person speaking it
salwar-kameez	Loose trousers and long shirt or tunic, traditionally worn by people of south and central Asia, and became popular in the southern India since the 1980s.
sari	A strip of unstitched cloth ranging from 4 to 9 metres in length (worn with a blouse) that is draped over the body in various styles by women in many parts of South Asia, Burma and Malaysia
tarawad mahima	reputation and honour of the joint family
Thalappoli	A traditional ceremonial procession by women or young girls in celebrations in Kerala to welcome God or honourable guests
Thali	A pendant made in gold worn by married women, also called *minnu* among Christians; its equivalent is *mangalsutr* in north India.
Thiruvathira	Dance form performed by women originally on the day of a festival with the same name
ulvili	Calling/strong inner urge
utsavam	Festival
uttara	Northern
Vamana	One of the ten incarnations of Vishnu as dwarf Brahmin
vayatatti	midwife

Vishnu	One of the three trinities of Hinduism responsible for the well-being of the universe
Yadava	A group of traditionally pastoral communities or castes in India and Nepal whose main occupation was cattle-raising and production of milk and milk-related items
yeh	This

Foreword

It is a matter of great pleasure for the Centre for Women's Development Studies (CWDS) that the work of one our faculty members, Sreelekha Nair, has been published. Several years ago, when the then Director of the centre, Narayan Banerjee, encouraged this study in its first stages, negligible research on the topic of nursing existed.

CWDS was established in 1980 as one of the first autonomous research centres in women's studies, and is supported by the Indian Council of Social Science Research (ICSSR), under the Ministry of Human Resource Development, Government of India. The centre is known for providing an enabling environment to ask neglected questions and to rigorously explore such issues, be it in the world of work, politics, health, or education.

Indeed, when one considers the subject of women and various professions, this study by Nair remains pioneering work in an area that demands much greater attention than it has received so far. This book brings to light how challenging it is to research and study this field. At the same time, it highlights the reward, of having contributed to this very significant area of research. While it is absolutely true that nursing in India is 'moving with the times', there is much that remains invisible. Recent years have undoubtedly witnessed a growing public interest in this profession, as well as a welcome involvement on the part of the nursing community itself in addressing its status and future. In that this is a timely publication. Moreover, even though the book explores the world of migrant nurses from the south Indian state of Kerala, recent studies on nursing from other parts of the world demonstrate how much is shared across disparate yet connected contexts and how much there is to learn. It is therefore hoped that this book will evoke as much interest in nursing in India, as beyond.

Mary E. John
Director
Centre for Women's Development Studies, New Delhi

Preface and Acknowledgements

It is indeed a great honour to have authored my first book. It is such a special feeling. And, that the subject is on Malayali nurses is not surprising in the least. I imagine that anyone sociologically inclined would be rather curious about them, their plans, work and movement from one hospital to another, from one city to another, and from one country to another very distant one. This book attempts to, at the least, partially fulfil the desire of many to know them better! Thanks to the Malayali nurses, especially the respondents and other participants in my research, who have made this possible!

I use this opportunity to reassure everyone who asked the question 'Why Malayali nurses?' that it has been worthwhile to study them. First and foremost, as a scholar interested in women and work, it appeared to me that nurses were conspicuous only in their absence in academic writings despite being the major single category of professional women who move in large numbers from Kerala seeking employment. Besides, they do generate interest— of course, not as potential subjects for 'serious' academic research but as women one encounters during a hospital visit. It is also true that the undercurrents and dynamics of women moving from the state of Kerala to the rest of India and beyond, the processes of their movement and their conditions of life in those places have not been thought upon as interesting enough. This book tells us through interviews with these women that their stories around these themes are indeed remarkable.

Questions of research methodology and its limitations when used within the strict boundaries of the discipline of one's training cropped ever so often, and one had to negotiate the path between presentations of experiences of the respondents in the study and the methodology employed to get to know those experiences. Engaging with the nurses who share common cultural and linguistic characteristics with me, in the city of Delhi where we all are migrants, broadened my horizons. Knowing more about them made me cautious about the way in which one interprets women's agency.

Interactions with the respondents introduced me to various issues of relevance in their lives—their self-perceived low status in their workplaces and society outside, the intense identity politics played out within the Malayali community in Delhi that centred on their gender and profession, and, of course, Delhi city as a springboard into their future. These are the issues that comprise the subject of this book. These issues also helped inform my approach and, therefore, the methodology of getting to know them better.

Centre for Women's Development Studies (CWDS), New Delhi, is the place that made me realise the plan to work on nurses. I owe a singular debt of gratitude to its directors—Narayan Bannerjee and Mary E. John—who supported every effort of mine and even pushed me to make this project a success. Kumud Sharma and all other colleagues at CWDS need special mention for the extensive and intensive discussions I had with them at various points of my research.

Anju Vyas, Ratna, Deepa, Vijay and others at the CWDS library were always ready to help with any query on available resources. Without Sundaresh's ever helping hand with computers, this project would not have been what it is. I also thank the libraries of Centre for Development Studies, Trivandrum, Queen's Medical Centre, Nottingham, Maison des sciences de l'homme, Paris, for the readings I had during various phases of this project.

I have collaborated with Madelaine Healey and Marie Percot—two scholars whom I admire—during the course of my research for this book and I thank both for broadening my perspective and for making me part of meaningful collaborations.

Discussions with various scholars and activists at different points have made this research an unforgettable experience. I must thank Marie Percot, Mary E. John, Mala Khullar, and the anonymous reviewer for all suggestions that have been invaluable for the book and for the broader understanding of concepts, issues and presentation of data. Various seminars and conferences sharpened my understanding of nurses and nursing, and I thank all those who were gracious enough to engage me on my research topic at various forums.

Last but not the least; I thank the Routledge India team for their cooperation and professional handling of this book.

Needless to point out, any failing that this book possesses is my responsibility.

FIGURE 1.1
Real and Imagined Migration Paths of Malayali Nurses

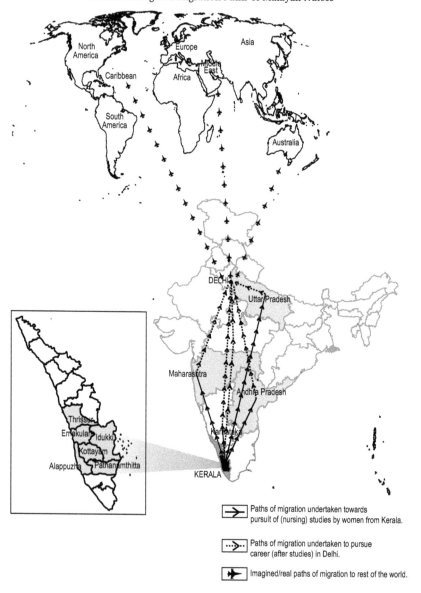

Paths of migration undertaken towards pursuit of (nursing) studies by women from Kerala.

Paths of migration undertaken to pursue career (after studies) in Delhi.

Imagined/real paths of migration to rest of the world.

Source: Prepared by the author. Map not to scale.

Introduction

The presence of large numbers of nurses from Kerala in every nook and corner of India, and indeed across the globe, frequently evokes the curiosity of the general public and figures in random discussions. Everyone at one point or another has seen or been served by a nurse from Kerala, or been in a hospital 'full of Malayali nurses'. Yet, in spite of their widespread presence, these nurses seldom appear in academic debates. The 'phenomenon of the nursing boom in Kerala' has been explained away without any serious attempt to document their lives, either as migrant women workers or as providers of health care, by pointing to the prominence that the state achieved in the development literature as an 'alternate model',[1] evidence of Kerala women's higher levels of literacy and health status.

It is not just Malayali nurses who are omnipresent and yet invisible. Indian nursing itself is absent, both in the existing scholarship and in the concerns of the Indian women's movement. This is the case despite nursing being a profession dominated by women. As a consequence, figures like Muthulakshmi Reddy, Haimavati Sen and Anandibai Joshi—all of them doctors—steal the limelight as pioneer Indian women professionals, whereas the names of pioneering nurses in India, or the names of Margaret Dean and Reena Bose,[2] who served the nursing profession for more than 50 years, are not part of any academic discourses or activist memoirs.[3] The women's movement has thus forgotten[4] its less illustrious daughters, exposing its own urban bias and exclusions, despite all the efforts that have gone into unearthing the worlds of women and work across the centuries to the present.[5]

It is precisely the image of being 'unworthy' of academic research and serious engagement that leads to responses such as: 'Yes, your stories are fascinating. You should write something "semi-academic" about nursing and nurses'. It is disheartening to read about those who studied nursing elsewhere, like Shula

Marks (1994: 1) who encountered its uninteresting, 'taken for granted and virtually invisible' status in the history of South Africa. This means that the most important point to state at the outset is the lack of literature and even basic data, which limits any discussion on the issue.

Apart from the rather random comparative descriptions found in discussions of occupational roles (Oommen 1978), nurses have recently found a place as subjects in the academic literature as migrants, with the new focus on international migration to countries in the North. International migration has received attention from academics and policy makers because, as R. Skeldon (2003: 3) points out, it is affected by national labour markets and macroeconomic processes in both the home and host countries. Concerns about transnational migration have started to show up in studies on nurses as a professional group in the context of globalisation and liberalisation.[6] S. George (2005) and M. Percot (2005, 2006) have explored the gender and class dimensions in nurses' transnational migration, throwing considerable light on the dilemmas, ambivalences and contradictions of nurse emigrants in the settings of the United States and West Asia, respectively. More in the nature of ethnographies and anthropological explorations, their studies mirror how families define themselves and get defined in exercising the choices of pursuing a profession that includes the experience of migration. Interestingly, it becomes evident that the new constructions of marriage that N. Kabeer (2007) recently discussed in the context of the emerging crisis in social reproduction and the global economy are, after all, not that new in the case of nurses. The gender role expectations from men and their masculinities have also been going through changes and the resultant predicaments have been illustrated by S. George (2005) and Gallo (2008), for example. The dynamics of race in the host country add further questions about the 'dreams at the destination' of nurse migrants.

The present study explores the most neglected dimensions of the world of nursing, namely, its status and dynamics within India. It does so by studying the life strategies of nurses from Kerala in the city of Delhi. I am particularly interested in frameworks that attend to the small acts of women in their everyday lives even as they negotiate national and transnational spaces and powerful social structures. Nurses' stories reveal numerous acts of resistance and defiance which, while by no means extraordinary, do have the potential to transform their world into a more egalitarian and less hierarchical place to live. Nurses' stories highlight the importance of recognising the need to engage with the system, however exploitative it might be, in the absence of any sight of a 'revolution' in the near future. Thus, women's agency is looked at as significant. Going beyond older structure versus agency debates, this study makes it amply evident that it is the complex interrelations between women's actions and choices and their structural contexts that must be accounted for. Quite in line with the findings of L. Fruzzetti and S. Tenhunen (2006: xiii–xv), women's actions can be quite paradoxical in their effects.

The migration of nurses from Kerala to different parts of the country has been a process to reckon with since the 1960s in terms of absolute numbers and proportions.[7] Focussing on nurses working in several Delhi hospitals, the following pages explore the critical roles of gender and status in the personal and professional experiences of my respondents. I further attempt to weave in the specific ethnic category of being a Malayali in Delhi, to map the lived realities of this particular professional group in the nation's capital. As this study hopes to demonstrate, to be a Malayali nurse is to constantly negotiate one's life and future at the intersections of gender, status and migration.

Nurses in this study challenge the hypothesis put forward by the push-pull demographic models of the 1970s and 1980s, where migration was seen as the outcome of individual decisions. Their movements are not captured by standard data-gathering instruments as they do not necessarily follow a linear pattern and involve more complex rural-to-urban and urban-to-urban circular movements.[8] As Percot (2006) has pointed out, Malayali nurses' lives are intertwined with those of their extended families at home in Kerala wherever they go. And this makes the migration process qualitatively different from those migrants who take a linear migration path of 'no return'.

Curious though it may seem, nurses are invisible in Kerala as well, carrying with their professional identity a certain banality because 'there is a nurse in every household'. This is only one of the many contradictions that the once-celebrated 'Kerala model' must now contend with—the low work participation rates of women, and the high levels of domestic violence—thus making the much talked about emancipated 'Kerala women an enigma'.[9] Unhealthy patterns of gender relations place high levels of stress on the lives of women, including mental health problems that have only recently received some attention.[10] Kerala's type of economic development, despite its laudable achievements in literacy, education and health, has been betrayed by its extremely low industrialisation and employment generation. In the context of the land reforms in the 1960s and the high population pressure on agricultural land, comparatively better educated youth migrated to various parts of India and the world beyond in search of work. Women nurses, mainly from lower middle-class and poor Christian families, composed one of these migrating segments.

The role of the family is evident in their migration experiences, though to different degrees, and not always as a solid block of support, as we will see later in this study. Paradoxically, sometimes the sheer inability of parents to guide their children has led to the decision to take up nursing and the concomitant need to migrate. In whatever form, family is in the minds of these nurses in the present and in their plans for the future. Thus, the rational individual is not completely absent but is shaped by the economic calculations of the collective called the family. Unlike early approaches to gender and migration, the responsibilities of women as wives and mothers (and the role of men as breadwinners) did not have a straightforward relationship to women's life strategies in this study.

Of the Field, Sample and Methods

'...but it is silly to imagine that you should (or could) 'enter the field' with a blank mind'. (Goldbart and Hustler 2005: 18)

The problem and the perspectives

This book began as a field-based study of Malayali women nurses' work and mobility as women in their own right, prompted by the large number of single women travelling in trains from Kerala to different parts of the country. While engaging with the experiences and viewpoints of such women, my initial interactions gave me the sense of a choate and powerful identity politics among migrants and the gender dynamics within the community. This then led to the unearthing of power differentials among Malayali working women (such as school teachers, computer operators, secretarial staff and accountants in private and public sector institutions) within the community, as well as non-working, married women. But within these, what stood apart was the marked status of the nurse in relation to everyone else. These layers of power have ossified through the creation and maintenance of the stereotype of the Malayali nurse which, in turn, structures the migrant Malayali communities' imaginations of the home that has been left behind. Their lives follow a migratory path through the discourses and debates on the status of their profession, seemingly wading through the ethnic and linguistic identity politics of the communities that make up the Indian republic. This politics is experienced often as isolated and one-time incidents that nevertheless leave deep impressions in their minds, and capturing them as they were described by the respondents and representing them here in order to give a 'wholeness' to the picture of their lives has been one of the greatest challenges of this book.

There lies a gulf between their lives and realities on the one hand and sociology on the other, notwithstanding the obvious possibilities of application of sociological theory and tools to understand nursing and nurses. This gulf is due to a number of reasons: the most important seems to be the fact that nursing is understood as work where nurses need to possess practical skills, and have knowledge of some basic anatomy, physiology and pathology. Moreover, we largely follow the 'biomedical' model of health and sickness and health is largely seen as a purely physical matter. Max Weber's notion of status that directly links occupation and educational attainment (Weber 1994: 125) comes close to a framework that may be useful to examine nursing and nurses' situation. More importantly, in support of using the framework developed by Weber to study nurses I would say that his analysis of social stratification has built up a sociological approach to the study of professions.

That is not to ignore the relevant critique offered by A. Witz (1992), that theories on professions do not take into account the reality of gender. 'The generic concept of profession is also a gendered one. It takes what are in fact the successful professional projects of class-privileged, male actors at a particular point in history to be the paradigmatic case of profession' (ibid: 64). Agreeing with her in this aspect of analysis of theories on professions, I want to make it clear at the outset that the marking of the nurse cannot be explained either in terms of class categories alone, or by market situation; it requires an exploration into the special history of nursing, the gendered nature of the hierarchy of professions in which it is entrenched, and its status anxiety. And in order to do that I have used a number of theoretical streams, including historical analysis of the profession of nursing and therefore use of the historical method is an important part of the analysis presented in the book.

Nurses are educated beyond secondary school. And yet, in spite of being 'well educated' in the Indian context, given the very low levels of general access to higher education in India, this does not translate into a corresponding level of status, as later chapters will explore more closely. Upward educational mobility, and even economic mobility, alone does not assure nurses of the socially valuable position they want. Looking at it through Weber's lens helps us understand that social honour is social in nature and does not mechanically result from a market or property relationship, but is an expression of social relationships. It can be associated with either positive or negative quality that is socially valued or is undesirable. Thus, even the near universal employability of nurses, which is a positive market situation, does not give them the social honour that they desire. As D. Grusky (1994) argues, status exists in a close relationship with the material domain, but is not determined by it. In the literature on the subject, status has often been seen to revolve around the ascription of honour and the sharing of 'special styles of life' (ibid.: 19–20).

As I discovered in the course of my research, the problematic status of the nurse needs to be understood as much within the organisational structure of the hospitals as in the relationships of these primarily single migrant women to the local patriarchal communities in the city and to migrants from other parts of India as well. Also, quite in line with the analysis of A. Abbott (1988: x–xii), the status anxiety of nurses mentioned earlier is relative and inevitable and is part of the manner in which professions negotiate their jurisdictional boundaries and social division of labour. Thus, the class and market situations, gender and status questions within and beyond the hospital complicated my initial sense of the 'simple and docile' Malayali nurses' existence in Delhi. While it is therefore necessary to press beyond the binary of a male-female experience of migration and work, gender powerfully mediates the experiences of these women and the multiplicity of their identities as professionals and as Malayalis in their everyday lives. One might speak of how nursing—as education and occupation—becomes a life strategy rather than merely a source of livelihood for the women in my study.

The field, methodology and the methods

The hospitals, hostels and homes of nurses in Delhi constitute my 'field' where I went about interviewing the respondents[11], studying their working conditions and observing their inter-actions with the 'significant others' in their professional and per-sonal lives. They work in different hospitals and nursing homes in the city. Delhi's health sector is extremely heterogeneous, and is broadly divided into private and government hospitals. In the private sector, recently established chain hospitals run by inter-national agencies, which have come up with the onset of liber-alisation policies, are large multi-speciality hospitals with approximately 500 beds, registered as private limited companies and trusts. The second category in the private sector consists of medium-sized hospitals and nursing homes with 150 beds. Third are the small nursing homes with up to 10–15 beds, though in some cases no in-patient facilities are available. Government hospitals are organised at the primary, secondary and tertiary levels[12] with similar in-patient facilities. The nurses I interviewed came from this wide variety of workplaces, excluding the primary health centres in the public sector. Personal contacts, snowballing techniques and then the sheer chance of being at the right place at the right time to start a conversation earned me the privilege of meeting more than 150 Malayali nurses. They were interviewed with the help of structured questionnaires apart from in-depth discussions. When I conceptualised the study, main objectives included looking at the working conditions of Malayali nurses in Delhi hospitals, which were often unfavourable, as I had gathered from the nurses themselves, and the processes of their migration from Kerala to the national capital of India. With these objectives in mind, I collected information on the types and nature of hospitals by searching for the secondary literature on them, including regulations of hospitals from the Directorate of Health and by visiting the hospitals. Initially the idea was to have a representative sample from all districts of Delhi. However it was soon realised that hospitals were not distributed uniformly across Delhi and some districts had clusters of same types of hospitals while some other areas did not have those types of hospitals. At the time, corporate hospitals, for example, were coming up in the south of the city while the other parts of the city had no such hospitals. Variations in the nature of the hospitals in the private sector itself were ample reason for the random selection of respondents. Difficulty in getting them to talk without a reference also proved difficult. So the sample is heavily dependent on the snowballing technique, as mentioned. The initial survey of hospitals was used to get in touch with the administration and to see whether there were familiar faces in the hospital administration or among the workforce, including doctors, to get permission[13], which often was the first step towards sitting down to talk to the nurses. Nurses with whom a rapport was built during this period were also helpful later on in introducing other nurses for interviews. What I want to emphasise is the importance of having a reference to set the ball rolling. A number of nurses and administrative staff helped me obtain formal permission to enter the hospitals. In a few cases, I was shown the door even in the middle of interviews.

Also relevant to mention in this context is the importance of the references nurses made in passing about certain incidents in their lives during the initial stages of my meetings with them that gave insight into the issues relevant to their lives in Delhi. These were sometimes repeated during my visits for interviews. These visits also helped me interpret the stray incidents described by the nurses as having powerful meanings in their lives, not to be dismissed as rare and/or exceptional. This in turn led me to include many of their stories—that sounded 'once in a lifetime' and critical—that had a powerful bearing on their lives in my research, thereby supporting the relevance of traditional anthropological fieldwork techniques that did not exclude any information that the researcher got in formal interviews and in other informal situations. Thus, this study looks at nurses' world from a social constructionist standpoint informed by feminist epistemology. This situates this study as one that is better understood by its objectives and not so much defined by its methodology. At the time I conducted my research, it appeared that an effort had to be made to make sense of nurses and their lives in their own words and through their own stories. Therefore, much beyond the analysis of the questionnaires, it is the stories and isolated incidents described by the nurses as significant that have found their way into this book. Observation of public lives and discussions with random people who could be engaged in a conversation on nurses provided important clues about nurses' images and how they were perceived and were talked about by others, much to the discomfort of the disciplinary and methodological rigour.

As can be seen from the table in Appendix, nurses of this study range from fresh diploma holders to degree holders in nursing, to Auxiliary Nurse-Midwife (ANM) who do all the work that a professionally trained 'nurse' is supposed to do. There are also respondents like Kavya, who had no training in nursing or any related field till she joined a private sector hospital with 15 beds a few months ago, and Lallymol, who has had training as a lab technician but that does not entitle her to work as a nurse as she has been doing in Delhi. Working in both public and private sector hospitals as staff nurses, vested with the duty to look after patients in wards, ICUs and operation theatres, this sample consists of nurses in the age group of 22 years, who had recently completed their nursing studies. This sample is skewed in favour of young nurses with 125 of them being below or at the age of 30. The remainder were above 30 years of age, the oldest being 51 years old. The sample was drawn mainly from hospitals in the private sector, 125 of them working in private hospitals of small, medium and large segments that mirror the organisation of hospitals in the health sector of Delhi.

The sampling technique depended on snowballing and availability of nurses for interviews and, hence, the sample of this study does not really represent the estimated 7,500 Malayali nurses in Delhi. The hospitals where the nurses were employed are spread across different districts of Delhi and reflect the general conditions of work and status of nurses in Delhi. The number of Malayali nurses is also greater in the private sector than in the public sector hospitals in Delhi, and an initial survey and observation of the hospitals for the study revealed that recent recruitments to public sector hospitals include fewer Malayali nurses.

Learning about them has been a very enriching experience, deepening my understanding of the multilayered existence of the 'empowered' and modern woman whose life tends to assume a clichéd meaning globally.

I also had the opportunity to interact with non-Malayali nurses, nurse leaders, doctors, administrators and some patients. Some of them were official 'gatekeepers' who held power to provide or withhold information and permission to facilitate my meeting with nurses. Participant observation in traditional festivals of the Malayali community in Delhi, interactions with patients at an informal level, discussions with non-Malayali neighbours on ethnic and linguistic issues in everyday lives in the neighbourhoods of Delhi, meetings with nurse leadership—at the professional association (Trained Nurses Association of India) and the Delhi Nurses' Union—who were non-Malayalis at the time of my interactions structured and shaped the study in unforeseen ways. Hospital administrators—almost always medical doctors at senior levels—were rather strict about granting permission for me to do the interviews in the hospital wards and surroundings. And yet a few of them openly expressed their opinion and views about nurses and nursing with requests not to quote them or to keep them anonymous.

It was practically impossible to list and tabulate all the information and data collected on nurses and their numerous sources, as every opinion and view helped and directed me to the exploration of the aspects discussed in this book. The last chapter on diasporic politics and identity is an attempt to put together these pieces of stories and information in order to give the reader a sense of the wide range of views expressed, that in turn are part of the experiences of the migrant nurses in Delhi. Though not substantive in the book, these voices are methodologically useful to scrape together the context of nurses' lives in Delhi. However, this part of the book is not to be understood by the methodology it uses but more by the assistance it offers in understanding the lives of nurses.

My own identity as a Malayali woman living in Delhi—albeit as a researcher—has undoubtedly shaped this study. Given the rich sociological and feminist literature on issues of subjectivity and objectivity in fieldwork, I was acutely aware of the interplay between 'empathy' and critical distance structuring my interactions at every step. Empathy was evidently in abundance, given our shared cultural, linguistic and migratory contexts, and was essential in our verbal and often non-verbal means of communication to build the trust to discuss personal lives. I also recognise that such empathy can itself be seen as objective and social, in so far as it is reflexively acquired through methodological training in sociological research.[14]

And yet entering the field and negotiating access to the experiences of nurses was not easy at any level. The respondent–researcher relationship was built on mutual perceptions about the shared context of the 'home' that is Kerala, as well as the internal hierarchies and micro-politics of the immigrant community in a metropolitan city. The boundaries of this study—indeed, the very experiences considered worthwhile—have equally been determined by my respondents. As D. Smith has pointed out in a different context:

> When you are committed to discovering how things are being put together, you can make discoveries that overturn what you took for granted and thought you knew. From such discoveries, more is learned about that institutional complex of the ruling relations than the researcher had known how to ask at the outset. (Smith 2007: 415)

My fieldwork yielded rich insights into nursing as a feminine sector of employment, and how patriarchal, class and status ideologies and practices define the local forms of this profession to a non-nurse. In India these are historically intertwined with colonial history, its institutions and contradictions. These dimensions will be contextualised in the chapters that follow.

Kerala women's dominant presence in the nursing profession in India as a whole cannot be explained without looking at the historical reasons why nursing became the accepted occupation for an increasing number of women from that particular state. Changes in agricultural patterns and land reforms which forced lower-middle class families to look for other avenues of income, and low levels of industrialisation in the state resulting in a stagnant rate of employment generation,[15] form the structural background where a developing modern hospital system and institutional nursing created new job opportunities. The early spread of education in Kerala, especially among Christians who embraced the new education system more quickly than the rest of the population, supplied these establishments with their first trainees. Nursing was definitely viewed as an escape from poverty for families and individuals. Less well known are the high levels of dowry prevalent in Kerala at the time of a woman's marriage, especially among Christians who display a particularly blatant form of patrifocal lineage. P. Kodoth has termed dowry as 'marking a radical transformation of marriage', as it occupies an important place in marriage transactions in a state 'better known for its development experience and matrilineal traditions' (2007: 1). At the same time, discourses of modern nursing at the time of India's independence created a space for those women who needed a source of income, without visibly threatening men's occupational ambitions. This, in turn, also provided breathing space for women from oppressive social norms (Nair and Percot 2007). It is by taking all these contradictory aspects into account that I have come to see nursing as a 'life strategy' and not a simple choice of a livelihood.

Practices of patrifocality in Kerala include segregation between men and women[16] and the ongoing low status of care work even when certain indicators of Kerala's better social development became visible. These advancements in terms of conventional indicators are important because they point to a minimum level of physical standard of living and life chances that the people of Kerala have. These are reflected in the better health and individual dignity that people in Kerala possess (Jeffrey 1992: xi; Kurien 1995)[17] compared to the rest of India. As Kurien points out, one important though not sufficient manifestation and cause of this advancement is public action and pressurising the state from below by different communities that organised themselves for the state to start and maintain welfare measures.

Migration

Meanwhile, migration—for women as well as men—to urban centres within India and abroad gained momentum as an alternative to the lack of employment opportunities in Kerala[18] (Zachariah et al. 2003: 14). Internal migration has been crucially important for Malayalis. According to Zachariah et al., '(U)ntil very recently, Kerala was known more for its internal (within India) migration than for its external migration' (ibid: 386). Two distinct periods are important in the migration scenario for Kerala. Till the 1940s Kerala was a net in-migration state. Subsequently, it became a state where the outmigrating population outnumbered the inmigrating one. This changeover came when educated, employable youth from Kerala got themselves employed in military and other civilian services after Kerala was integrated with other states in the Indian Union. According to Zachariah et al. this started with the Second World War. 'The number of persons from Kerala moving to Chennai, Mumbai, Kolkata, Delhi and other metropolitan centres exceeded the number who came to Kerala from other states' (ibid.), thus making the region a net outmigration space. This en bloc movement as far as numbers are concerned, albeit as a collection of individuals, was first to different Indian cities from the 1960s[19] and then to the Persian Gulf, the US and the UK. Delhi, the field of our study on migrant nurses, is regarded as a non-traditional destination. Migration to this city started long after the movement to other places in the south and west had been established (ibid.: 45).

This takes us to the point where the question has to be reversed. Rather than asking why so many nurses come from Kerala, we need to locate nurses within the field of the highly gendered and class-differentiated 'model' and pattern of development in Kerala which manifested 'a central tendency and an outlier'[20] (Kurien 1995). Due to their heterogeneity, women come from the centre as well as the periphery, given their different socio-economic and caste-class backgrounds. Considering their vulnerability as single women workers migrating to another city, nurses occupy the peripheries in the patriarchal social world of Kerala.

In internal and international contexts, the strategies and mechanisms of women and men are diverse, having been shaped by their gendered social situations (Nair and Percot 2007: 8–31). The problems that confront women migrants are qualitatively different from those faced by men, even at their destinations, due to patriarchal structures. While female migration is substantial, the value attached to both the migrations and expectations from the migrants by Kerala society are not the same. Indeed, academic debate around migration in Kerala has only recently acknowledged the gender dimension of the massive outmigration from that region (see, for example, Zachariah and Rajan 2004). When a man migrates and finds employment, it is seen as success, especially if he is able to demonstrate his affluence through conspicuous consumption at home[21], in the form of acquiring land and constructing a house in particular. But the equivalent is not true for women. This is not to say that the successful migration of women is not socially appreciated. The status and self-perception of women, however, seem to suffer and the discourse in this case revolves around ideal feminine attributes. Appropriate gender role expectations seem to catch up with women who take the migration path, thereby enforcing a double burden on women who must go through the demanding processes of relocation and acclimatisation. For example, Gallo (2008: 180–212) points out that pressure and expectations to marry at the 'appropriate age' and the rumours around their prolonged absence from home lead women migrants to maintain an ambivalent relationship with their community and family in Kerala.

The opening up of labour markets outside India and the processes of globalisation have brought opportunities for nurses to work abroad and earn considerably more than is possible in India; further, the deflation of the Indian rupee against the major currencies of the world favours international migrants. Working conditions are also better in the technologically superior hospitals of rich countries. International migration is thus seen as the solution both to unemployment in Kerala and the lack of satisfactory working conditions in the hospitals of the country.

The mass emigration of nursing professionals, however, leaves already ailing Indian hospitals with a shortage of trained nurses and, thereby, exacerbates an already poor nurse-patient ratio. It also slackens the collective pressure on improving the working conditions through collective bargaining, as women keep shifting their place of work. Little attention has been paid either to the working conditions in most Indian hospitals or to the nature of the demand for Indian nurses abroad. In effect, while large numbers of women seek to emigrate, their life strategy follows an individual trajectory, once again preventing the development of collective forms of bargaining as carers and pro-fessionals for the many nurses who continue to work in hospitals in the country. As M. Burawoy (2000: 1–35) points out in connection with a discussion on the academic possibilities of a 'global ethnography', studying the experiences of these Malayali nurses makes the links between global and local processes palpable. Even though my fieldwork was restricted to the city of Delhi, it was continuously connected to Kerala, the Persian Gulf, US, Ireland and other foreign destinations through the lives of the nurses. Thus Malayali nurses' experiences, plans and imagined futures evoked multiple sites. Equally visible and relevant in their lives are the all-powerful modern states, ever-vigilant about national identities and the privileges of their own citizens, especially when labour is crossing over from 'less advanced countries'.

Migration is not a simple movement from one place to another, but a complex set of experiences for the nurses who are in constant engagement with the space they have left behind. In a number of cases, coming to Delhi is not the beginning of their journey. In such cases, the move beyond Kerala begins with plans to study nursing, which takes place at a stage in their lives when young women are dependent on family members or kin. Delhi marks a phase in their lives as they search for economic independence, even as emotional ties and other forms of family dependence continue. Many of my respondents displayed a contradictory mix of claiming new freedoms in the city away from home, while eager to show that they were dutiful daughters and sisters who would never cross the '*lakshman rekha*'[22] or do anything that would malign the family and its honour. A few could provide a more nuanced picture of how family ties depend as much on economic considerations as on emotional ties. Their discourse on independence, career, freedom and personhood has clearly been conditioned by the highly patrifocal Malayali nuclear family, which, in turn, both as an instrument and as an end in itself, is at the centre of contemporary development. This 'modern family', with its strictly defined gender roles, is essentially a monogamous, middle-class nuclear family whose conservative codes of sexual morality are promoted by prominent community organisations, church and political parties alike.

The construction of the two-fold model of '*ghar* (home) and *bahar* (outside)'—the domestic and the public spaces—which was part of the cultural project of the nationalist movement[23] and was also sustained by the established left politics in Kerala failed to question the domestication of women's space inside the home and the lack of access to the public spheres that characterised Kerala's modernity. 'The absence of a recognized position attesting to women's contribution to society and the nation left voiceless women in an invisible space' (Fruzzetti 2006: 11). This had the concomitant effect of leaving unquestioned men's role within the domestic space. In spite of a strong left movement, Kerala society has thus internalised a powerful private and public dichotomy rather than exploring progressive or innovative ways of undermining it. As Fruzzetti argues, ghar has been rigidly defined by kinship identities, thus leaving no space for women and other vulnerable groups to negotiate public spaces, including that of politics (ibid.: 1–20).

While issues of gender and migration have been studied in other contexts in relation to the family (for example, Pedraza 1991), attention in India remains relatively recent (Thapan 2005). In the context of Kerala with its longer history of emigration, most of the debate was concerned with men who 'are the migrants and actors', while women are the passive recipients of the men's actions. Migration surveys were undertaken without including women at any stage, even when they were active participants in the processes of migration of male members and their families (Gulati 1993, 1997). Thus, a neutral, 'ungendered' image of migration—which, for all practical purposes, was highly masculine—evolved in academic research. Only later, in response to such critiques, were women tacked on to existing frameworks. It is thus only recently that migration studies have benefited from perspectives that are sensitive to women's differential experiences.

Women's contribution to national and family economy is inevitably associated with feminised[24] sectors of employment (Ghosh 2004: 17–19; Kukreja 1995). The new literature on feminisation has also highlighted the preference for young girls between the ages of 16 and 23 in certain sectors of employment for their perceived suitability due to their 'nimble fingers' and compliant outlook. This preference for young women has also been linked to 'push' factors due to transformations in agriculture and the attractions of the city (Deere and Leal 1981). In the present study, migration of workers, especially women, has been precipitated by a combination of diminishing economic opportunities in rural areas and perceived opportunities for urban employment, contributing to the relative urbanisation of the female population (Kukreja 1995: 19). Relatively higher proportions of secondary education among women, relative female urbanisation, and low agricultural productivity have thus been offered as the most significant variables to account for new patterns of migration among women in the literature. However, issues of status, much less those of empowerment and autonomy, with which this study of the nursing profession is centrally concerned, have not been adequately foregrounded in this literature.

Improved professionalisation has been seen as a panacea for the status problems of practitioners of modern professions in various discussions in sociology (Madan et al. 1980; Oommen 1978). Sociological approaches to professionalisation try to link them with years of training and autonomy. Oommen (1978), for example, found that lack of professionalisation and the salient character of its work milieu were responsible for its erosion in a profession like nursing. But there are other arguments that nursing has been professionalised at the expense of autonomy. Hawker (1987: 147–50) examined the loss of autonomy in the hospital system in England and its consequences for patients and their families. She explores how nurses are accounted as part of the hospital's 'cost', whereas doctors and other professionals are seen as the opposite. Thus, doctors add to the reputation of hospitals, whereas nurses' dedication and professionalism seem to have no consequences for the hospitals' standing. If nurses are good service providers that fact is generally understood as given and at best it is something that is said in passing by the patients, and only among themselves. It is clear from the limited accounts on nurses that there is more to nursing history and practices than labour history. Writings on nurses agree in general on one point: that nursing has been reformed and is developing towards the modern profession that everyone seems to want it to be. Different perspectives in the scholarship on nursing and its history have to do as much with gender and class relationships as about acknowledging nursing's inferior position within medicine in the 19th century and the pace of growth of the profession.

Existing studies also reflect a relative power struggle within health care. C. Maggs puts this power struggle rather simplistically as follows:

> Doctors urgently needed more nurses to meet the demands they were creating as medicine expanded and preferred to develop training programmes which would produce competent nurses as quickly as possible. Nurse leaders wanted to educate nurses, not just to train them; they favoured a more systematic and structured approach to nurse education. (1987: 3)

Considerable documentation of the struggles of leaders like Nightingale is available. But what is missing are the links between nursing, its 'low' status and women's social position, on the one hand, and with working class and trade union movements and professional organisations, on the other. An unusual example is the nurses' movement in France where they succeeded to some extent in linking the above issues, though the profession there too is plagued with many of the ills seen elsewhere (Kergoat et al. 1992). Hierarchies within the profession, as in the case of Indian nursing, led to a lack of collective bargaining, while male-dominated trade unions failed to take into account the interests of women-majority occupations.

The present debates on globalisation make visible the complexities that arise in a context where individual opportunities and success stories are defined and given focus without looking at the asymmetries in global power that come from links with the colonial period. Competition and assertions of ethnic and national identities have also challenged the idea of a globalised world. Yet, it is difficult to discount the importance of migration to the 'other world' in the lives of nurses and other professionals. Indian nurses' life strategies are deeply structured by the reinforcing effects of poor working conditions at home and the attractions of better opportunities elsewhere. The constant comparison between options available 'here' and better possibilities 'elsewhere' makes the present situation look grimmer than before. This is why the internal migration of nurses in the country is linked to the dynamics of international migration and cannot be understood from a national perspective alone. As P. Sharpe says '...a revolution in transport and communications, and the increasing disparity between earnings in rich and poor countries, makes a 'transnational' existence far more common than has been the case before' (2001: 2).

The media, both print and electronic, contribute to the prevailing perceptions of women's work and migration in general. Nurses are sparsely represented, whether in employment or in migration coverage. Nurses are newsworthy at the national level only when there are sensational cases of rape and violence or a rare national strike. Nurses (like Manjulata whom I interviewed as an activist of DNU) who have been part of the Delhi Nurses' Union for a long time, however, feel that the degree of negative reporting in the press, over which the Union issued frequent protests, has decreased over the years.

In the context of Kerala, it is migration to the Gulf that is covered most frequently, considering that over 2,500,000 Keralites work there. Changes in residence rules in the Gulf and declining job opportunities are thus of maximum interest as more Malayalis are forced to return home.[25]

This study goes beyond standard approaches in sociology in approaching nursing as a profession. It is not just that I approach questions of professionalism more broadly, but also that I have chosen to follow the experiences and perspectives offered by the respondents themselves. I have also benefited from the more recent approaches of feminist ethnography and sociology in openly adopting a partial standpoint as a researcher who cannot be disengaged from the subject of my research. In the process, my identities as a feminist, a Malayali and a migrant have surely played their part. However, as theorists like S. Harding (1993: 49–82) have argued, a reflexive approach that includes both the researcher and the researched is potentially more objective than an objectivist stance that denies the observer any role. As a 'true' sociologist, therefore, I have tried to look at my 'self' critically and cultivated the necessary critical distance from my subjects as well. Nonetheless, at this stage of my development as a sociologist, I believe that it is necessary to privilege the intersubjective realm of knowledge creation in order to substantiate the interpretations of nursing that I am about to offer.

This study is organised into five chapters, an Introduction and a Conclusion. The development of nursing as a modern profession in the context of India and Kerala is explored in Chapter 1. Understanding nursing in Kerala in the context of its evolution as a province of the Indian federal system and its colonial and princely state inheritance, this chapter helps contextualise the factors that led to the educational choices of nurses in the study. It is a prelude to the discussion on the status of nursing, the subject of Chapter 2, which presents the experiences of nurses regarding their status in their professional lives. Chapter 3 examines the processes of opting for nursing as a profession, as a life strategy, that encompasses both themselves and their families. Choosing nursing is the first step of a life plan that has migration woven into it as the next logical step. The multiple dimensions of migration in Delhi, as a stop along the way, form the subject of Chapter 4. Chapter 5 stages the professional, linguistic, ethnic and cultural dynamics of the migrants' life vis-à-vis the local population, as Malayali women bargaining with the social norms of the migrant community and Delhi's localities and neighbourhoods. The concluding chapter ties the study together.

Notes

1. Discussion on Kerala's development (or lack of it) and its nature springs up every now and then, considering the centrality of the social and physical space of Kerala in the lives of the participants of this study.
2. They were among the 17 awardees given the Nightingale Award for nursing personnel in 2007. The award was reconstituted that year, after a gap of 18 years.
3. In Geraldine Forbes' chapter (2005a: 79–100) titled 'Managing Midwifery in India', the discussion on midwifery revolves around the contributions of missionaries, memsahibs and Indian modernisers, especially the women doctors of the early colonial period. This speaks volumes on the way nursing leadership is perceived by those outside nursing, and also the invisibility of the nurse leaders themselves in written documents. Nurse leaders were not recognised as women whose agency was instrumental in the development of nursing itself.

4. Urvashi Butalia pointed out in a discussion that it is not that the women's movement forgot the nurses' cause but that it was ambivalent towards the nurses' movement. Her point is well taken, but in effect the result has been indifference to nurses and nurses' issues within the women's movement.

5. See Forbes (1996: 155–58) for an understanding of the vagueness of the discourse on women and work in colonial India.

6. Even then, nurses as a group of migrants attract the attention of only women sociologists. At most, they appear as numbers in economists' estimates of skilled migration (see, for example, Khadria 2007).

7. But their movement is not taken seriously by researchers, possibly due to the 'mundane and uninteresting' nature of the whole topic (as mentioned earlier), or because women's migration lacks importance in the agenda of documenting population movements, and is perceived as 'having no economic consequence'.

8. See Skeldon (2003: 3) for a discussion on the difficulties of measuring these types of movements.

9. See Mukhopadhyay (2007: 3–31) for an interesting discussion.

10. Mukhopadhyay et al. (2007: 86) write that the '[s]tatus of mental health problems improves with higher levels of education, the impact is more pronounced for men than for women. In fact for women, the education variable is not significant before one crosses the level of secondary education'.

11. Though I prefer the word participant, it is debatable whether one can use the term 'participants' in studies like mine where one is hardly able to make them participate in the research beyond the period of collection of information. Time and financial resources as well as the concept of research in academics do not allow any room for the participation of the people about whom one writes. Nevertheless, the terms *informant* and *respondent* do not reflect the intentions of the research either, though, in effect, they remain at the level of respondents to the researchers' questions in the present state of scientific research.

12. See http://delhigovt.nic.in/dept/health/hospital.asp for details.

13. I am indebted to Dr Sumit of a prestigious hospital in central Delhi for my first formal interview of a nurse with the questionnaire. Thereafter, contacts worked much more easily and nurses started introducing me to other nurses, making me travel from the north to the east and then to the south and to the west, eventually back to central Delhi.

14. In this context it is interesting to look at the discussion by Smith (1989: 44–48) on 'Designing Objectivity: Emile Durkheim and Others'. She discusses how Durkheim brings in the social as the

agent and how one's own subjectivities as a researcher are shaped by sociocultural contexts and, therefore, are objective in a certain sense (pp. 39–41).

15. This employment scene is mainly about men who were the 'breadwinners' and the lack of opportunities for them in Kerala. Hence, there was a need for women to enter work outside the domestic space.

16. Refer to Mukhopadhyay (2007: 175–79) for images of this seclusion of gender in the public space, both religious and secular. George (2005) too talks about this in the context of the church service on Sundays in the new destination in the United States.

17. 'The public action measures that this government (the first communist government of 1957) initiated in the agrarian sector, such as land reforms, abolition of tenancy, granting of homestead rights, ensuring of minimum wages and the improvement of working conditions gave a fillip to the physical conditions of life and created a great upsurge and assertion of self-respect and dignity among the vast masses of the agricultural labourers and small peasants in Kerala' (Kurien 1995: 72).

18. Kerala was reported as a net in-migration state during British rule though the Second World War seemed to change that. Recruitment of Malayalis as soldiers, civilian clerks and military officers along with the abolition of slavery elsewhere seemed to have broken this trend.

19. Chandrakanthi, member, Kerala Medical Council, gave me a clear picture of the starting point of nurses' migration, which was supported by others who discussed this subject. She puts the 1960's as the starting point of nurses' migration from Kerala.

20. The Kerala model has been criticised for its differential developmental effects on different communities. Some communities benefited marginally, while others were the main beneficiaries.

21. Filippo Osella and Caroline Osella (2000) nail it down to a more complex phenomenon than described here. There are various stereotypes that represent men migrants, depending on the nature of their show of affluence and monetary success.

22. This literally means 'Lakshman's line' and means a limit that you cannot cross. In the Ramayana, Ravana abducts Sita once she crosses the line drawn by Lakshman, her younger brother-in-law. Though Lakshman is inferior to Sita in status due to this relationship, by virtue of being the man he is attributed with greater wisdom and worldly knowledge, which Sita, being a woman, seems to have lacked.

23. Chatterjee (1994b: 121) maintains that this ghar-bahar dichotomy came to be identified through the social roles of gender. While answering the questions on women, he argues that the nationalist

paradigm did not reject western modernity in its entirety but rather selected what suited its project. For a discussion of the colonial engendering in the region of Kerala, see especially the work of J. Devika. Devika (2007), for example, discusses in her thesis on the language of reform in early 20th-century Kerala that men and women came to be seen as belonging to separate social domains—the public and the domestic—having different kinds of endowments. About the women's question in the nationalist movement in the world in general, Forbes argues that '(t)here is a general agreement in the historical literature that a women's rights movement does not easily fit with a nationalist movement…when women insist that redress for their grievances be given higher priority than the national struggle, they will be considered subversive' (1981: 51). However, the Indian nationalist movement was an exception, she argues, as social reformers of the 19th century concentrated on women's status. Nevertheless, as Mazumdar (1990: 54) points out, though the dignity and status of women within the family got some attention, economic and legal independence of women beyond their roles as wives and mothers received little support from most social reformers and nationalists.

24. Here, 'feminised sector' is used as an almost equivalent of feminine and is intended to mean, in this context, that nursing is a women-dominated profession. Because care work has historically been a woman's domain, women are not actually replacing men in their jobs, or women are not new in nursing, but they are still in the ghettoes as far as this sector of employment is concerned. As the discussion progresses it becomes clear that being a women-dominated profession has contributed towards the neglect of nursing by policy makers and administrators, causing it to remain a low-status occupation globally since its inception.

25. *The Hindu*, 19 August 2008, p. 7.

1

Beyond Well-being

Development of Nursing as a Modern Profession in Kerala

Development of nursing as a modern[1] profession in Kerala is intertwined with the integration of Kerala society and economy with the global (read 'imperial') plans for development, on the one hand, and the evolution of it as an independent political unit that joined the Indian Union, on the other. The role of the state and Christian missions along with the involvement of people in broad policy measures have been a characteristic of Kerala's development experiences (Nair 1998; Tharakan 1984). Princely states like Thiruvithamkoor (Travancore) and Cochin are documented to have played a very active role in the development of literacy and health of their people. Ever since the Thiruvithamkoor-Kochi and Malabar regions of the British Madras Presidency came together to form Kerala as a state based on the policy of linguistic reunification of states in 1956, various governments have focused on social sector development, including that of health (Oommen 1999; Tharakan 1984). The following section outlines the emergence of nursing in Kerala within the context of the growth of modern nursing in the world as well as the dominance of the western model of caregiving, despite the existence of traditional private nurses and midwives called *pettachi* or *vayatatti* in Kerala.[2]

Along with this are issues related to the contributions of missions and charitable and health research foundations. The fact that early conversion and spread of Christianity in Kerala predates missionary activity in the field of health and education, as discussed by Meera Abraham in her introduction[3] (1996: vii), is often overlooked. Nevertheless, considering that nursing, as a modern profession, was inseparable from the religious orders of different Christian denominations, the association of Christianity with nursing is not all that ill-founded. Prominent models of nursing that shaped Indian nursing, such as the Nightingale model, did emphasise the religious nature of the profession (George 2005: 41). However, for the majority of the nurses in my sample, nursing was an occupation more than a calling. Some of them define it in terms of spiritual acts of 'doing good', rather than in religious terms. Yet, there are reports of nurses refusing to be part of abortions out of the compulsions of their faith.[4] Most importantly, in the beginning there were so few nurses that recruitment efforts had to focus on women who needed economic means for survival. C.B. Firth points out that 'around the period of the Second World War, 90 per cent of Indian nurses were Christians, and 80 per cent of Christian Indian nurses were trained in mission hospitals'.[5]

When Indian sources are discussed, Susruta (widely believed to have lived between 1000–600 BC) and Charaka (lived between 3–2 BC) are often mentioned.[6] They talk about patients' attendants in ancient India and these can be imagined only as non-specialised, male disciples of physicians. Knowledge of drug preparation, shrewdness, devotion to patients, and purity of mind and body are described as the qualities of the attendants. There is no room for logical deduction of the existence of women nurses though. Buddhist monks constructed hostels where they kept the sick and the deformed for cure and care (Wilkinson 2001: 5). The decline of Buddhist power in political circles also led to the decline of these hospitals, and priest physicians of the Brahminical order were not in favour of any physical contact with pathological tissues, fluids and body parts.

Wet nurses and women who are specialised in attending to births are mentioned in various accounts on social lives across the world (Sarasúa 2001). Wars and religious orders have contributed to the development of nursing as an organised vocation. Christian orders emerged as nursing specialists. Women were given admission to these orders 'because service to cattle and to sick persons' was better performed by women (Bullough and Bullough 1978: 41). Mendicants who concentrated on the nursing of the sick and the wounded, like the Franciscans and Carmelites, travelled far and wide to reach the poor and the needy. Imitating Jesus' life was more a concern than the nursing itself (ibid.).

Thus these religious origins of nurses contributed to the image of nursing as a calling and duty, as also to the word 'sister'[7] to denote a nurse. The difference between nurses and people who nursed their relatives was that the latter were neither regulated by any statute nor were they responsible practitioners of care. Nurses' duties included keeping records of those whom they nursed, making beds, washing the patients and the clothes and adhering to the cleanliness norms for themselves. Images of femininity and ideas of good women became associated with their ability to nurse the sick. A strict watch was kept on these nurses by their supervisors to see that they did not mingle with men at odd hours, and did not remain idle or do other work. In short, strict discipline, unquestioning obedience to physicians' orders, seclusion from men, and devotion and warmth towards patients were features of the western model of Nightingale nursing which formed the basis of Indian nursing.

Many women seemed to have gone beyond simple nursing duties to assume the responsibility associated with modern nursing and all midwifery work appears to have been done by women (Bullough and Bullough 1978). Nursing care remained within the family, especially the female members. Unlike the medical sciences and physicians, nursing and nurses were never part of broader inventions and innovations that came from changes in scientific temperament and religious beliefs and superstitions. The end of the 18th century marked the beginning of important reforms in nursing in Europe, along with huge urban growth. This seemed to be the period when nurses' salaries and the status of nursing were discussed in connection with hospital abuses. This period in nursing history is significant as it marks the shift of nursing from the private domain to the public domain, caused by the need to care for the masses wounded in the wars. In fact, Nightingale's contribution, most importantly lies in the institutionalisation of patient care. Nightingale's argument for a respectable salary for nurses was presented as part of the concern for patient care. At that time, nurses held a degrading position, probably because of the low status of women in the patrifocal set-up and because it was not proper for women from 'respectable' families to enter nursing. It was only the guise of religious motivation that allowed women to enter a profession like nursing where the work included touching the body fluids of strangers, including men.

The secularisation of nursing and the admission of the masses to nursing invariably led to 'lower-class' recruitments in Britain from the Crimean War period, that is, mid-19th century, and after. The unmarried, the widows and the destitute—all in all, the outcasts—had to work to earn a living and respectability was of secondary concern. Low pay, long hours of care, night work, and the degrading public attitude towards nursing stopped many women of 'good families' from entering the profession despite their concern for the sick. The moral values of the time prevented women from entering even educational institutions beyond the preliminary level, let alone nursing. Nurses were generally looked upon as paupers, and their deprivation, which was reflected in their food and clothing, led to an image of nurses as careless, sloppy old women, very much like Mrs Gamb and Mrs Prig in Charles Dickens' stories.

It is only the sanctified image of Florence Nightingale that could shake the indifference that the well-to-do and middle class felt and showed towards nurses and nursing. This apathy was a major hurdle and, in fact, continues to be so for the founding of secular, organised nursing. Nightingale's entry into nursing helped the image of nursing in England because of her wealthy background, political influence and domineering disciplinary routine with nurses. Even in India, the image of Nightingale as the 'lady with the lamp' helped nurses find a clear path of action for themselves and continues to do so even now.[8] She was able to bend the rules and limits with her perseverance and influence during the Crimean War. She became the strong yet compassionate, ever-sacrificing ideal of womanhood. She transformed the image of nurses as noble and valuable, published 'Notes on Nursing' (1859) meant for the average housewife and 'Notes on Hospitals' (1859) arguing for better management of hospitals. Her efforts for trained nurses met with stiff resistance from medical authorities and doctors who were afraid that nurses, once trained, could become a threat to their profession (Bullough and Bullough 1978). She had to resort to the typical 'patriarchal bargain'—the tactic of projecting women as 'feeble, weak and ladylike', who cannot do much without the help of 'strong and powerful' men. Women candidates had to conform to the likeable image of a nurse as a competent mother or a wife who cared for the sick, an image which persists till today. Due to the spread of the British colonial empire to different continents, nursing throughout the world was based on the British model and the contribution of Nightingale nurses was high everywhere, including in India. This is not to ignore the valid criticism by many who worked on nursing history that the Nightingale experiment was exaggerated to mean something more than what it actually was and was 'ossified as tradition'.[9]

The first official nursing school was established by Florence Nightingale and Sarah Elizabeth Wardroper, with the help of Sidney Herbert (Secretary of War and Nightingale fund), at St Thomas Hospital in London in 1860.[10] Supervision and elaborate character assessment in terms of discipline, trustworthiness, personal neatness, good character, and morality more than the cognitive aspects of education became the focus of the Nightingale model of nursing (Baly 1987; Bullough and Bullough 1978). Going by the experiences in the Crimean War and related events, they concluded that working-class girls were the best for the experiment. Probationers had to move in pairs and were chaperoned to stop them from getting lured into the 'temptations of the world'. These were seen as measures to 'raise nursing from the sink'. A hierarchy was in built within this model as women from better-class backgrounds[11] were special probationers who paid for their board and lodging, were given more medical lectures than the regular probationers and worked in the hospital for only two years. Regular probationers were paid a small stipend and had to work for three years for a nominal wage after their probationary period. Selection, education and hierarchy were independent of the medical system but were strictly under the order of doctors when they practised their care of patients.

Thus, the submission of nursing to medical supervision and the ideal caring woman as a modern nurse have their origin in this model of nursing which became the dominant influence in nursing in the erstwhile British colonies. This model considerably influenced Indian nursing also due to Nightingale's association with India as a member of the Royal Sanitary Commission on the Health of the Army in India. Her expert comments on the Indian situation do not in the least bit betray the fact that she never visited India.[12] She criticised the Indian hospital system for its lack of comfort, shortage of infrastructure facilities and lack of dedication. Her interests included concerns to raise the sanitary levels in military hospitals, and later in civilian hospitals and the overall health of Indians in general. By 1868, her efforts bore fruit and many reforms in the British Army in India were implemented and a sanitary department in India was created. Nurses who were trained in the Nightingale Nursing School came to India.

Development of Nursing in India

The influences of the existing nursing model—the Nightingale model[13]—and the modifications for each region affected the growth and the shape of nursing, and India was no exception. The growth and expansion of the hospital system in the West also necessitated the growth of nursing as a profession in India. Imperial colonisers who came to India like the Portuguese, the French and the British contributed to an established order for nursing. Due to their long stay in India, the British had to take into account the long-term interests of their troops and the general conditions in India. This facilitated the establishment of a medical system and nursing. The East India Company founded the first civil hospital for soldiers in Madras in 1664, which later became the Government General Hospital. A nursing training centre was started in 1859 in Calcutta by the Government of Bengal to make trained nurses available. The National Association for Supplying Female Medical Aid to the Women of India, under the initiative of Lady Dufferin, took the first step on a national scale towards serious intervention in nursing in 1885. It was only in 1888 that the foundation of Indian Army Nursing was laid in Bombay.

British colonial efforts in organising care professionals for the Indian Forces, which were vital to fight imperial wars across the globe, consolidated the system of modern nursing in India. Civil and mission efforts for better nursing service helped include the masses in the nursing profession, both as receivers and as givers of care. The First World War (1914–18) compelled the British to initiate measures to supply caregivers and nurses for the army but these were not regular policies aimed at developing a regular supply of nurses. Such a measure would have needed educational policies and institutions, which were clearly lacking in India. Nevertheless, nurses were recruited for the first time for the Queen Alexandria's Military Nursing Service for India in 1914. The Indian Military Nursing Service was born during the First World War and was described as such in 1927. Three years' training in nursing was started in select military hospitals, and when the students became registered nurses after passing the final state examinations, they were commissioned as members of the Indian Military Nursing Service. This state of affairs is understood, from scanty sources, to have continued till the Second World War (1939–45), which necessitated the expansion of the Indian Military Nursing Service, literally on a war footing. Due to the abysmal shortage of trained nurses, the Auxiliary Nursing Service was established in 1942.[14] The ad hoc nature of the constitution of the Auxiliary Nursing Service is reflected in its form even now. It provided six months' training in select civil hospitals and then sent the trainees to serve the army as assistant nurses.

Civil and mission hospitals brought nursing to the masses and to the reach of the public beyond the war and the soldier. Nursing's lack of mass appeal could be detected even before this period. However, the stark disparity between the demand and supply of nurses started when the number of hospitals expanded. Apart from the status issues that plagued nursing, norms of seclusion, ideal womanhood and defined domesticity of women and, to some extent, the preference for Christians and those who had religious training similar to those of the missions were reasons why recruits hailed from certain sections of society. Anglo-Indians and Europeans formed the majority of nurses, mainly due to their higher educational levels compared to the very low educational levels of the general population. Low status, lack of educational facilities, and poor living and working conditions were cited as reasons for the lack of interest by 'suitable girls' (Nagpal 2001a: 23). To improve the situation, grants were sanctioned, mainly by the Dufferin Fund[15] till it handed over all its hospitals to the Government of India in 1947. Grants were given to select hospitals to build nurses' hostels, supply teaching equipment to training schools, employ trained nurses in hospitals, and send trained nurses for administrative training abroad. Significantly, the mission hospitals were the first to recruit Indians as nurses.

Policies regarding the individual status of persons who were to become nurses are not directly available in the literature except that caste, class and gender factors determined women's entry into any field. Women were required to show that they were single or legally divorced to join nursing. However, there are some references to married nurses joining the local wing of the Indian Military Nursing Service in 1958 (Wilkinson 2001: 15). They had to have three to five years of training experience and be a registered nurse and midwife between the ages of 21 and 35. 1968 and 1996 were critical years in military nursing, when the law governing the married status of nurses in the military service was reformed (Wilkinson 2001). Prior to 1968, Nursing Officers had to resign their commission when they got married; due to the shortage of unmarried nurses, pragmatic changes were made and marriage was no longer a disabling factor for the career advancement of military nurses.[16]

Efforts were made to train traditional *dais* and integrate them with nurses-cum-midwives in order to meet the demands for nurses in the expanding health care system (Nagpal 2001b: 62–63). One important measure emphasised by nurse educators to standardise and professionalise nursing in India was the need to register existing dais and midwives. This also seemed to have resulted partly from the colonial policy of discounting indigenous midwifery practices as 'unscientific', which later led to critiques of these measures as ethnocentric and biased. Anshu Malhotra (2003: 229–60) has described how the British officers' assault on traditional dais 'revolved around their purportedly 'dirty' habits, lack of formal training and the unhygienic conditions of childbirth'. From the perspective of the colonial administrators, the dais posed a serious threat to the reorganisation of midwifery and the latter resisted the schemes meant to integrate them with the new system (Forbes 2005a: 95–96).

The present-day Trained Nurses' Association of India came into existence as the Association of Nursing Superintendents in 1905 at Lucknow. The organisation was established and run by nine European nurses holding administrative posts in hospitals (Dhaulta 2001: 210). There were attempts to standardise the norms and practices of nursing classes, syllabi and the medium of instruction in various regions between 1907 and 1909. This was also the period when a large number of foreign nurses were reported in India, mainly as matrons and nursing super-intendents (Nagpal 2001a: 24). One example of regularisation and standardisation was the North India United Board of Examiners for Missions Hospitals, which was formed by a Conference of Nursing and Medical Superintendents. This body was joined by their counterparts from the government and Dufferin hospitals. Similarly, in the Madras Presidency, which included the present Indian states of Tamil Nadu, parts of Karnataka, Kerala and Andhra Pradesh, a Nursing Committee of the South India Medical Association was formed. They met to decide on the conduct of nursing courses in the hospitals of the region and a uniform for the nurses.

Indian State and Nursing Post 1947

Nursing education, nursing services and public health nursing are the three major aspects of nursing that developed in India after independence. Public health nursing has been used in India to reach out to people and bridge the gap that existed (and continues to exist) between the majority of Indians and modern health care structures. Major innovations were undertaken for the existing colonial models and practices. This section concentrates on the policy measures and interventions made by the Indian state. These policy measures have to be seen in the context of the state and the status of nursing at the time of independence, as well as the fact that the ratio of nurses to the population was completely unsatisfactory. Another important consequence for the nursing profession was the cementing of its subordination within the medical profession which was already in-built in its inherited form as a western profession.

In its efforts to improve the medical system in general, the Indian state set up different committees, and implemented some resolutions and guidelines provided by international agencies like the World Health Organization (WHO), International Labour Organization (ILO), and UNICEF. The International Council of Nurses (ICN)[17], in particular, guided nursing leaders and the government on various issues. The Government of India appointed a number of high-powered committees to survey health care services and to suggest remedies. The first committee, set up in 1943, produced a document with recommendations that remain relevant and unimplemented even today.

(i) Committees

1. **Bhore Committee (1943–46).** This 'Health Survey and Development Committee' under the chairpersonship of Sir Joseph Bhore was to (a) conduct a broad appraisal of the health conditions and health organisations in British India, and (b) suggest measures for the growth of modern hospitals in India.

   The committee confined itself to the period up to 1941 in its report. It looked at all aspects of health services and studied the organisations of the medical, nursing and public health services at the local levels. It recommended very important steps, such as the organisation of village health committees and national health organisation and services. The following are the fundamental recommendations of the committee that were relevant to the nursing profession and services at that time.

   (a) **Regulation of the nursing profession**. The committee recommended immediate regulation and standardisation of the nursing curriculum and practices, including those of midwives and health visitors across British India. For this purpose, it suggested an All-India Nursing Council that would co-ordinate the activities of the provincial councils and assist in laying down minimum standards and safeguarding them.

   (b) **Increase in the number of nurses**. It was estimated that the total number of registered nurses was around 7,000 (Nagpal 2001b: 62). The committee recognised the importance of raising the number of trained nurses. A public health nursing service for preventive and curative work in India was essential and more people could be attracted only if the conditions of nursing improved.

   (c) **Improvement in training facilities**. Preliminary training schools were to be established which would give elementary instruction. Junior Grade Nursing Certificate Programmes and Senior Grade Nursing Certificate Programmes were suggested, depending on the educational qualifications of the applicants and the number of years of training in the course. Middle school was the required educational qualification for the junior grade and matriculation for the senior grade.

(d) **Stipends for medical and nursing students.** To facilitate the entry of large numbers of students from all economic and social backgrounds, a monthly stipend of ₹60 to half the students was recommended. This amount was to be recovered from them in instalments.

2. **The Shetty Committee (1954).** The Government of India appointed a committee on the advice of the Central Council of Health under the chairpersonship of A.B. Shetty, the Minister of Health of the state of Madras.[18] The importance of this committee lies in its special focus on the nursing profession. Ms Adranwala, the then Member Secretary of the committee, was the nursing in-charge of the Directorate of Health at the central level. The mandate of the committee was to look into both education and practices in nursing, as well as to report on the gap between existing requirements for nurses and their availability.

This committee also emphasised the huge shortage of nurses and suggested reforms in training patterns and the status of nursing. By now the status problem in nursing had been explicitly pointed out and the need to attract girls from 'good families' was highlighted. Existing service conditions and emoluments were found inadequate and uniform salary scales and other conditions were recommended across the country. Some recommendations suggested providing residential facilities at the hospitals for student nurses and teaching wards in hospitals. The nurse-patient ratio in hospitals with nursing schools was fixed at 1:3 and in hospitals without student nurses at 1:5. One health visitor was to serve 100,000 people. The committee also recommended a larger teaching staff and a reduced administrative load for matrons and ward sisters so that they could concentrate on their nursing duties.

3. **Mudaliar Committee (1959–1961).** A 'Health Survey and Planning Committee' was set up by the Ministry of Health, Government of India, under the chairpersonship of Dr A. L. Mudaliar. The terms of reference for this committee were to examine developments in the health sector after

the recommendations of the Bhore Committee and to formulate further health programmes from the third Five-Year Plan (1961–66) onwards. Nursing was only a part of the committee's area of concern and its recommendations regarding nursing reiterated those of the earlier committees. The committee recommended three grades of nurses: general nurses (four years of training and matriculation as the minimum educational qualification), auxiliary nurse-cum-midwife (two years of training) and graduate nurses (higher secondary or pre-university as the basic educational requirement). As a transition step, it suggested relaxing the age criterion for admission in regions where girls were not coming forward to join nursing. English was suggested as the medium of instruction even for general nursing and English was compulsory for the graduate course.

Considering the difficult living and working conditions of the student nurses, the committee suggested measures to focus attention on their hospital training and practical learning. Free board and furnished lodging in the hospitals where they worked, free uniforms and laundry, free books and medical services and recreational facilities were to be given to the nurse students. Stipends were recommended at ₹35, to be increased by ₹10 every year. It must be noted, however, that the recommended increase in the number of nurses was ultimately meant to enable doctors to be released from the mundane work of the hospitals so that they could attend to 'higher levels' of their work.

4. **The Chadha Committee (1963)**. Also known as the Committee of Integration of Health Services, it focused on the integration of nursing services and grades. It also looked into the requirements of lower-grade nursing personnel and the need to integrate family planning measures with other health services and its delivery through multi-purpose health workers.

5. **Kartar Singh Committee**[19] **(1973)** or **Committee on Multipurpose Workers under the Health and Family Planning Programme**. Like the Chadha Committee, it stressed the need to integrate multipurpose health workers with the rest of the nursing service.

6. **The Shrivastava Committee (1975).** This committee advocated the development of voluntary and part-time community-based health workers. The Community Health Workers Scheme of 1977 was the outcome of this recommendation. This committee has also been called the Group on Medical Education and Support Manpower in some writings.
7. **The Bajaj Committee (1986).** As Table 1.1 mentions, the Committee's recommendations influenced the creation of health universities in different parts of India, including state-level universities that standardised courses, including nursing education, in different colleges.

TABLE 1.1

Committees on Health in India and their Major Recommendations

Committee	Major recommendations	Implication for nursing
Bhore Committee, 1946	Establishment of degree courses for nurses. Called for urgent measures to increase the doctor–nurse ratio.	Long-term implications; became the major basis for nursing reforms. But many of the suggestions were not implemented.
Vishwanathan, 1953	Measures for dealing with shortage of nurses	Measures taken but not adequate even until now.
Shetty Committee, 1954	Provided for the standardisation of nursing across India. Public health nursing was to be made part of nursing curriculum.	Appointed to look exclusively at nursing.
Mudaliar Committee, 1961	Stressed on grading and specialisations of nurses.	Had long-term implications for the hierarchy within nursing.
Chadha Committee, 1963	Integration of different nursing services.	Led to the development of basic health services.
Kartar Singh Committee, 1973	Advocated integration of health services.	—
Shrivastava Committee, 1975	Measures for the training of voluntary, part-time community-based workers.	Community health workers scheme during the Janata government was a direct outcome.
Bajaj Committee, 1986	Measures to increase the number of trained paramedical personnel and health-related vocational courses	A few health universities were established

Source: Reports of various committees.

The aforementioned committees were appointed by the Indian state with the intention to reform and improve the health sector, as seen in Table 1.1, and yet the implementation of various measures suggested by the committees and the progress in the sector in general, and the nursing profession in particular, are still incomplete. However, the discourse of the state and the practice at the ground level regarding the professionalisation of nursing and nurses lingered. There was a wide gap between the desired state of affairs and the implementation of these desires in terms of policies formulated by the Indian state before and after independence.

(ii) Indian Nursing Council (INC)[20] and State Nursing Councils

The Indian Nursing Council or INC was established in 1947 as a response to the Bhore Committee recommendations for an all-India body to supervise nursing standards. The INC brought about significant changes in the prevailing system of nursing education in 1950. General Nursing and Midwifery was regularised as a three-year course with nine months or more of midwifery, and Auxiliary-cum-Midwives (ANM) were to undergo two years' training. The minimum education for the former was fixed as matriculation and for the latter as seventh or eighth standard. Courses like the Junior Grade Nursing Certificate were replaced by the ANM. Nursing Councils exist at the state level, too. They are the regulatory bodies on nursing education, curriculum and institutions, thus giving or withdrawing recognition and putting up criteria for nursing courses.

Other Influences

American nursing and the Rockefeller Foundation in particular are interesting areas to look at while discussing the history of nursing in India and the various influences on it. The Rockefeller Foundation played an important role as a major philanthropic organisation during the 20th century. The foundation helped organise public health nursing as an extension of its growing interest in funding programmes of preventive medicine. Leaders of the Rockefeller Foundation, in their interventions in India, were clear that broad reforms in both nursing education and practice were required. The foundation identified the need for a university setting to train nurses and made this distinction clear vis-à-vis traditional hospital-based training programmes. Their efforts in this direction, however, were localised to Vellore in south India and Delhi in north India. In Thiruvithamkoor[21] the foundation confined itself to research on tropical diseases and training medical doctors (Kabir 2003). However, its contributions are well known, especially in the form of grants to establish the Christian Medical College (CMC) in Vellore and the Medical College in Thiruvananthapuram, Travancore-Kochi (Jeffrey 1992).

American nursing experts working with international organisations in India from the late-1940s into the mid-1960s played a role in shaping the direction of Indian nursing. The task of the Indian state after independence, after various recommendations by high-powered committees, was made difficult by social and economic realities at the ground level. Gender and class factors stood in the way of developing a modern, professional nursing system, modelled after the West[22] (Nair and Healey 2006). This led to the status problem in Indian nursing that persists to this day.

It was clear that nurses who were interested in Indian nursing at the international level wanted women from 'privileged' sections to join nursing. And the programmes they developed, including degree courses, were meant to get the 'status' issue out of Indian nursing by encouraging this section to join them. With the prevailing educational levels among women, only a few degree schools could be started in India through the 1950s and 1960s, with the main ones at Delhi and Vellore. USAID helped develop degree colleges in Hyderabad, Indore and Jaipur. Rockefeller's substantial involvement with the College of Nursing in Delhi faced several problems because of the low standards and constant staff shortages, apart from problems of the hierarchy within nursing. In this context, the contribution of American nurses and their leadership in the creation of infrastructure for university-based nurse education should be recognised.

The beginning of 'degree education created a problematic division between clinical nursing on the one hand, seen as the preserve of diploma trained nurses and administration and teaching, which were the province of the degree educated'

(Healey unpublished). This gave way, in fact, to the continued devaluation of nursing practices and staff nurses in the hospitals. Trained nurses with degrees become teachers or managers, often with the bare minimum of actual nursing experience—which persists even today—due to acute shortages in teaching and administration. Ward experience was devalued, while standards of teaching in particular were quite low.

Various committees and policy makers projected public health as an area where trained nurses would be involved as the main personnel; in this, they were influenced by American nurse leadership and practices in America. A major component of the nurses' professional assertion in the United States was their involvement in the arena of public health where they had carved out a strong and publicly recognised role for themselves. However, there were many factors in the Indian context that Indian policy makers as well as American nurses failed to recognise. Large infrastructure gaps between rural and urban areas in India were a disincentive for nurses to work in rural hospitals; this was exacerbated by the low status attached to nursing.

Independent fellowships for training abroad empowered a few professional leaders, who gained confidence from their high-level education. Most of them wanted to set up independent and autonomous nursing schools and to promote better stand-ards in nursing education. On the whole, these programmes pro-vided some teaching expertise during times of critical shortage.

To summarise, nursing in India as it exists and is practised is a colonial product. There were many traditional practices includ-ing that of midwives or dais but the nurses as we see them in hospitals are the result of India's engagement with the West as a colonised, 'less advanced' country. There were many influences and streams from western countries including the United States. Leadership looked towards the West for views and perspectives for its development and borrowed many ideas and practices.

Being the main instrument in national development, the efforts of the Indian state in developing a modern hospital sys-tem included setting up several committees to look into profes-sionalising nursing. This was in keeping with the model inherited from the British. Ethics, spiritual devotion typical of religious orders, middle-class education and working-class resoluteness were seen as the requirements for a good nurse. These qualities were part of the assumptions of the common man and the political leadership alike and these assumptions about nurses were carried to nursing in India. It was in this understanding of the Indian situation that we need to look at Kerala and its 'phenomenon of the nursing boom'.

Development of Nursing in Kerala

As Robin Jeffrey has pointed out, 'the development of nursing as a profession in Kerala provides a way of measuring both attitudes—particularly those involving women—and the spread of government investment in medical treatment' (1992: 193). However, one finds that (this considerable degree of) favourable attitudes towards women only partly explain the entry of many women into nursing in Kerala.[23] At the time, important structural changes were occurring in the economic and social spheres of a post-independent and unified Kerala as a result of its global linkages and their expansion.

Before going into the details of those aspects, we will look at developments in the health sector and nursing and midwifery in regions that later formed the present state of Kerala. Kerala was reorganised as a state in the Indian Union in 1956, with the three regions of Thiruvithamkoor, Kochi and Malabar that spoke Malayalam. The princely states of Thiruvithamkoor and Kochi were grouped into one state in 1949 and Malabar joined in 1956. In terms of state interventions and public responses, the three regions were therefore distinct (Nair 1998).[24]

Thiruvithamkoor was ahead of Kochi and Malabar with regard to the availability of western medical facilities and care at the beginning of the 20th century. The London Mission Hospital started to function as a small medical centre due to the efforts of a British doctor called Dr Ramsey in 1838 at Neyyoor and that might have been the first western attempt to build a 'modern' hospital in Thiruvithamkoor. In 1928, 30 hospitals, 38 dispensaries, 18 grant-in-aid medical institutions and 14 mission hospitals dispensed western medical care; this was even higher than in many British Indian provinces.[25] Vaccinations against small pox, typhoid and cholera were already available in Thiruvithamkoor. Here, public health interventions by the Rockefeller Foundation focused on research in tropical diseases and US trade interests guided the Foundation's activities around the world[26] (Kabir 2003).

The government of Thiruvithamkoor requested the foundation to help organise a public health department along 'modern lines' in 1928 and a positive response was conveyed after the functionaries of the foundation surveyed the area. 'High rates of literacy, wide circulation of newspapers, network of hospitals and trained medical personnel' were seen as suitable for the activities of the foundation (ibid.: 12). One of the main activities of the foundation in the region was the control of malaria and plague. The foundation specified that its activities would be limited to some areas of its interest such as the codification of public health law, public health education, training in public health, treatment of hookworm, malaria and filaria, and sanitary engineering and sanitation. But in 1929 a public health unit was incorporated in this plan. The Neyyatinkara health unit was set up in 1931 to include diagnosis and treatment of infectious diseases, midwifery services, school medical inspection, food and milk inspection, vaccination against small pox and typhoid, treatment of hookworm and malaria and study of epidemic diseases, supervision of latrine construction and collection of vital statistics (Kabir 2003). But as far as implementation was concerned, the interests of individuals at the helm of affairs often guided the priority areas of the foundation. This was reported as a major success.[27]

Midwives and public health nurses were trained in the health unit and also in similar health units in Ceylon. One midwife was appointed for each revenue village. Going by the available evidence there was nothing historically remarkable about Kerala that led to the later supply of a high number of nurses. '...before 1947, even in Travancore and Cochin, the number of Malayali nurses was not notably high' (Jeffrey 1992: 193). There were traditional 'pettachis' and 'vayatattis' who helped women with the delivery of children, and by the end of the 19th century there were irregular trainings conducted for midwives by hospitals. During Miss Hacker's period as Nursing Superintendent (1902–27), a nurses' training programme for men and women in Malayalam was initiated at the London Mission Hospital, Neyyoor (Kabir 2003). Standards were low, and in 1926 strict measures were taken to raise standards and to provide more intensive training. Later, teaching was started in Tamil and English to cater to the needs of others who came forward and to bring about uniformity among trainees.

The association of nursing with religiosity, religion and Christianity and the notion of a 'calling' in Kerala are not accidental. This probably is the unique characteristic of the development of nursing in Kerala. Nuns were associated with nursing and hospitals from the beginning in Thiruvithamkoor. The Catholic Order of Sisters of the Holy Cross from Switzerland was invited by the Maharaja of Thiruvithamkoor when Mary Poonen Lukose[28] was the Durbar Physician (Abraham 1996: 83). The Holy Cross sisters were originally known as the Institute of the Teaching Sisters of the Third Order of St Francis of Assisi, located in Menzigen, Switzerland. Benziger, Catholic Bishop of Kollam, solicited their presence in Kerala at the Maharaja's behest. The Bishop felt that 'a true sense of dedication counted much more than a diploma' and desired that they 'witness to Christ by living a life of poverty and simplicity'.[29] The first batch of eight nurse-nuns came in 1906 (Aravamudan 1975: 257). They were given a salary of ₹40 per sister, with an allowance of ₹10 for the superior, and free living quarters and servants. They were reported to have been unhappy with their living conditions despite the enthusiasm of the Bishop. Still, their discipline and knowledge of managing the hospital's everyday up-keep were valuable. In 1909 more came, and 'a few of them had some elementary training in nursing'. They were also given nursing classes by Dr Mary Poonen Lukose. Formal nursing courses were established in hospitals at Thiruvananthapuram and Ernakulam in the 1920s. By 1938 Thiruvithamkoor had 108 nurses of whom more than 50 were Europeans (Jeffrey 1992: 193). Moreover, dowry had become an integral part of Christian marriages because of which women from the middle class had to earn for their own marriages.

When the School of Nursing started in Thiruvananthapuram in 1943 (ibid.: 194), the Holy Cross Sisters were given charge of 'technical and practical training' (Abraham 1996: 84). The total intake was 50 students. A similar programme admitted 25 students at Ernakulam in the Kochi region (Jeffrey 1992: 194). The first nursing school in Malabar was opened at Kozhikode in 1958 by the communist-led government of Kerala. A Holy

Cross Sister was a member of the first Travancore Registration Council for nurses. They had sufficient specialised training to be involved in such tasks as teaching operation theatre work. The new Thiruvithamkoor-Kochi state had fewer than 400 nurses, most of whom were Malayalis (ibid.: 193). In 1956, the Indian Province of the Holy Cross Sisters had 79 sisters, of whom 57 were Europeans and 22 Indians. In 1958, the Holy Cross sisters were given permission to start a training school for auxiliary nursing midwives. At the moment their school also provides General Nursing-Midwifery or GNM training (Abraham 1996: 84).

In south India there were as many as 75 listed mission schools of nursing. In about 33, standards were reported to be low. This was defended by western nurses on the grounds that Higher Grade Certificate Courses required higher education standards, whereas Lower Grade Certificate courses were conducted in the vernacular. But influential nurses felt that there was a need for equalisation and regularisation (ibid.: 101).

The dominance of Christians and the high presence of Protestant Christians in the profession even now is a result of their monopolisation of schools and the reluctance of Hindu girls to enter the nursing profession (ibid.: 102). Early marriage was less frequent among Christians compared to Hindus and Muslims in the region and, therefore, the former were more available for higher education and professional training. There was a mixed trend among Christians with some sections still going by traditional practices with life rituals, whereas some families preferred to adapt to the 'progressive' models and practices preached by the European missionaries (Jeffrey 1992).

> Nursing, to be sure, seems to have carried slightly less stigma in Kerala than elsewhere in India, but until it was clear that a nurse found ready employment, families showed no enthusiasm for making their young women nurses. Increases in the number of nurses awaited the expansion of training facilities and the assurance of employment that resulted from the simultaneous expansion of health services. (Ibid.: 193)

Thus, it is clear that families were ready to send girls for nursing because of the financial contributions they could make after their nursing education. It was not the idea of 'liberating womanhood into the public space' that resulted in women coming out to take up nursing. The 1960s was an important period for the training of nurses in Kerala when, according to the information acquired through interviews, nursing started becoming more popular as a job. The need for a student nurse labour force became increasingly the reason for hospitals to start nursing schools attached to their hospitals leading to an increase in the number of nurses in the coming decades. Thus while the total number of nurses reported for the year 1961 was 933, for the year 1983 it was 4,894.[30]

The expansion in nursing job opportunities led to a greater supply of young women for nursing. It was a guaranteed form of employment where they could invest even if the pay was low. Looking at the class background of the women who joined nursing in the initial decades, Morrison's observation of a small village in Alappuzha (formerly Alleppey) district in the 1990s becomes relevant. '(T)he hopes for the future were focused on education and entry into a wider arena of income-earning opportunities, not on farming ...' (1997: 72) . Women's nursing did not need investment since they got a stipend to keep their expenses off the family budget.

Nursing, thus, had more to do with getting a job than a religious calling, although the association between religion and nursing is still very strong. Aravamudan concludes that 'hardly any...came because they wished to care for the sick. They came mostly because it was a job' (Aravamudan 1975: 255). The socioeconomic status of the families was such that jobs were needed 'even' for their women. Kerala was undergoing major transformations due to the Land Ceiling Act, and changes in social hierarchies (Namboodiripad 1984); agriculture had ceased to be a source of income for the lower middle class and even the poor. Cash crops became less income yielding with fluctuating demands from colonial countries. Education was seen as an alternative for a better life, both economically and socially. There was no organised opposition to women's education and health-seeking behaviour (Nair 1998; Tharakan 1984). Customs of dowry and disproportionate inheritance of parents' property due to patrilineal practices, particularly among Syrian Christians, made it difficult for many to manage without women working to earn their dowry. This was true of Christians among whom these traditions were very strong. The Travancore Christian Succession Law granted that 'a daughter shall inherit one fourth the share of a son or ₹5000.00 whichever is less' if the father died intestate (Roy 2005: 224). It was only in 1986 that this was replaced by the Indian Succession Act which entitles sons and daughters to an equal share[31] and one-third for the widow.

A similar situation existed even for women of other communities, including ones with matrilineal traditions like the Nairs. Changes in the family system through legislations without any alternate support system left women from these communities helpless.

> [W]ith the rapid division and alienation of property, the individual share of many ordinary women was next to nothing. Large scale pauperisation was a common feature of this period, and women were certainly bigger victims. The *tarawad*[32] which sheltered them withered away. For many women from the big landowners' families, the period under discussion offered many new opportunities—education, employment and even political participation—but life for women in the not so well to do *tarawads*, which were not only losing property by division and alienation, but were also strife-ridden by litigation and disharmony between members became suffocating. (Saradamoni 2005: 220)

Progressive policies attempted to provide relief to landless tillers and socially ostracised, ignored women who were tormented by various social inabilities. The Malabar Tenancy Act, 1951 and 1954, the Agrarian Relations Bill, 1959, and the reform measures of the 1960s and 1970s provided legal sanction to the protected and secondary role to which the *marumakkathayam* woman had been relegated since British rule and the ideology that accompanied that rule (ibid.). Institutionalisation of relations of power and privilege thus failed to take women into account in their programmes when education in many cases became the only way out due to the numerous sanctions on mobility. Despite this, Nair women and women from Hindu and Muslim sections of the Kerala population entered nursing in small numbers; the small numbers can be attributed to the inhibitions based on caste and social hierarchies and the image of nursing as polluting.

With the increasing demand, nursing schools started fee-paying courses, and there were nine government and 17 private nursing schools producing about 450 nurses a year by 1977, which increased to 84 private nursing schools with 840 fee-paying students (Jeffrey 1992: 194). The migration of nurses, even to places like Newfoundland and the Gulf region, became common and nurses' migration to different Indian cities was common by then. If all these conditions had not come together or co-existed along with a market for their services elsewhere, nursing would not have been so successful in Kerala.

We will end this discussion by trying to answer the question: How did Kerala become the state which produces so many nurses? The high population pressure on land in this tiny state increased with Kerala's land reforms. Agriculture ceased to be a sustainable means of livelihood for many. People caught up with modern education and literacy in Kerala at a higher rate than elsewhere in the country. The search for white-collar jobs became the driving force in the desire for social respectability. Job opportunities in the growing service sector elsewhere in India have played a crucial role in allowing the unemployed rural and urban population in Kerala to cope with the consequences of agrarian distress and lack of employment. This connection between investment in education as a strategy and migration should not be understated[33] in this context though mobile, working women have not been given visibility even in Kerala.

Nursing did not come to the public domain and popular imagination as an appropriate life strategy independent of these developments in Kerala society and economy. To quote Morrison (1997: 64): 'Many farmers were encouraging their children to seek occupations with more attractive life prospects. Farmers were also diversifying their own income earning opportunities out of agriculture.' Of course, it appears that nursing as a course for higher education and occupation received less resistance in Kerala, especially among the Syrian Christian community, in comparison with other regions in India.

Thus, investing in nursing looked logical and girls joined nursing education in large numbers, looking for employment. City hospitals in Mumbai and Delhi never failed to provide the nurses with employment; these pulled the young women look-ing for an independent means of living towards nursing. Since questioning women's morality and character when they step outside the domestic sphere seems to have been the norm in rural, patrifocal communities like Kerala, it is only the compulsions of class that made women choose nursing. Many like Mariamma and Parvathy in the sample chose nursing because it provided free training[34] and often carried a stipend[35], making it easier for them to decide and join the course without any help from the family.

We also have to keep in mind the horizon formed by structural facades in the educational and employment arena in Kerala. High rates of unemployment and one's own socio-economic location act as two powerful factors that constrain the course of action in the choice of subjects. The high levels of educated unemployment among women and men in Kerala and the nurses' position within the so-called lower middle class or even the poor, therefore, determined these women's major decisions. Nonetheless, it is to the credit of the progressive social policies of various governments in Kerala that women have access to minimum levels of education and primary health care in the state. This makes sure that, allowing for the capability of individual women, they are able to take decisions about their own livelihood and enter the space created by modern nursing.

Notes

1. 'Modern' here is used to mean recent and progressive, rather than western. This is not to deny the influence of the western (North) countries on the formation and development of nursing.

2. Pettachis, by definition, were birth attendants or women who help in parturition and come close to the *dais* of north India. They attended to the births and took part in post-partum care of the mother and post-natal care of the newborn. Though they were private nurses in the sense that they functioned independently, each villager and family had a right over her services. Folklore suggests that they were bound by a sense of moral duty to serve despite their own health or economic consideration at any time of day or night. To that extent they could command the villagers on certain issues, though their ritual status appears to have been low. Yet, their status was considerably better than the *chamar* dais in the Hindi belt. Nevertheless, Anshu Malhotra (2003: 231, 246–47) mentions that the traditional dai with all the limits on her person had some level of access to power and the powerful in local settings in north India, like in the Punjab. Dais, she argues, also shared a rather long lasting relationship with women of all castes; hence, the same dai was asked to help with all the deliveries of a woman and a household.

3. Christians in Kerala are believed to have converted in four major waves. First, apostle St Thomas is believed to have converted the Syrian Christians in A.D. 52 and this is accepted as an apocrypha and not a historical account in academic circles. St Francis Xavier is accounted as responsible for the conversion of the Latin Christians in the 16th century, marking the second wave of conversions. The Anglicans converted the Dalit Christians in the 19th century (the third wave), and 20th century witnessed the Catholic denomination of the Syrians (fourth wave) (http://abrahamtharakanblog.blogspot. com/2007/07/history-of-conversions-to-christianity.html).

4. This issue has been discussed off and on internationally and in India. For example, see Worldnet Daily, 23 July 2009 and 'Catholic nurses ordered to help with abortion', *Times of India*, 19 December 2006 and Wajihuddin, Mohammed. 2006. 'When nurses are Muslims', http://articles.timesofindia.indiatimes.com/2006-12-17/india/27813741_1_nursing-school-muslim-girls-profession.

5. Firth (1960: 202) cited in George (2005: 227).

6. See, for instance, Wilkinson (2001: 1-7).

7. In the early years, 'sister' referred to a nurse who supervised the ward and the nurses worked under her. Slowly, a hierarchy evolved in a descending order of matron, sister, nurse, helper and watcher.

8. India's highest national honour for nursing personnel is called the National Florence Nightingale Award for Nursing Personnel. It is given to selected nurses on 12 May, International Nurses Day, by the President of India. It was revived after a gap of 18 years in 2007 during the tenure of President A.P.J. Abdul Kalam. Honouring Ms Alamelu Venketaraman as the awardee on 12 May 2008, President Pratibha Patil described 'gentleness, compassion and sensitivity as the innate qualities of a woman ... as a result of which she (a woman) dominated the nursing profession' (*The Hindu*, 13 May 2008, p. 10).

9. Nightingale herself was cautious in her approach to the first experiment in St Thomas Hospital, London, and said 'we must proceed slowly and by experiment'. See Baly (1987) for more on this and also the bargain between the Nightingale Fund and St Thomas Hospital.

10. Wardroper was the matron of St Thomas and became the head and manager of the School of Nursing. Sidney Herbert was the Secretary of War during the Crimean War and was an old friend of Florence Nightingale.

11. Women who came from better economic and social backgrounds put their motivation to join nursing as 'religious call'.

12. Nightingale sent detailed questionnaires to all military stations in India apart from obtaining regulations relating to health, sanitary

arrangements and administration. She wrote individually to each military officer of high rank. She secured figures on mortality, sickness, number of invalids in the army, length of service of invalids, and arrangements of barrack accommodation, etc.

13. Swiss nurses contributed much towards developing organised nursing care in the princely state of Thiruvithamkoor, as discussed in the section on development of nursing in Kerala.

14. All these measures led to a tangible hierarchy within Indian nursing, contributing to its adverse status.

15. Forbes points out that The Countess of Dufferin Fund or more accurately the National Association for Supplying Female Medical Aid to the Women of India is treated as the first of the series of endeavours towards a co-ordinated effort for western medical care for Indian women. At its beginning, the Fund states its objectives as 'providing medical tuition to doctors, hospital assistants, nurses and midwives; medical relief through dispensaries, female wards, female doctors and female hospitals; and training nurses and midwives' (2005a: 86).

16. Many nursing training institutions deny admission to married women and impose criteria based on marital status and physical requirements (*The Hindu*, 25 November 2005). The Nursing and Midwives Act, 1947, states that only women who are unmarried, legally divorced or widowed can apply for a nursing course. A particular height and weight were prescribed as part of the eligibility criteria. This act was amended in 1986. According to the above report, when asked a question in the Rajya Sabha by a Minister of Parliament (MP) from Kerala, the then health minister, Anbumani Ramadoss, directed the states and nursing councils not to impose any discriminatory eligibility. However, pregnancy and maternity remain major obstacles for nurses, especially in the private sector, in pursuing an uninterrupted career. Many nursing schools still have an informal policy of admitting only unmarried women as students (interview with Mrs Mattoo, Principal, Apollo Indraprastha School of Nursing, New Delhi, December 2008).

17. The International Council of Nurses is a federation of national nurses' associations (NNAs), founded in 1899, representing nurses in more than 128 countries. Founded in 1899, ICN is the world's first and widest-reaching international organisation for health professionals (as claimed in its website). India's affiliation as a member country was earlier withdrawn due to issues on membership fees. However, india has again become a member of ICN in 2011.

18. After India's independence in 1947, Madras Presidency was reconstituted as Madras state.

19. Between the Chadha Committee and the Kartar Singh Committee, there are two other committees: the Mukherjee Committee (1965 and 1966) and the Jungalwalla Committee (1967). However, their recommendations had little to offer the nursing sector.

20. The headquarters of the INC are situated in the Combined Medical Councils building at Kotla Mubarakpur in New Delhi. The INC supervises the standards of the nursing curriculum and they decide to update the curriculum. Their publications include the syllabi of various courses in the nursing schools and colleges of India.

21. The princely state of Thiruvithamkoor or Travancore was one of the three parts of Kerala that were united to become the present state in the federal arrangement of the Indian Republic in 1956.

22. See the chapter titled 'Status of Nursing: The Sword of Democles?' for a detailed discussion.

23. As we will subsequently explain, the need for women to find their own dowry led many women to nursing. This is neither liberating nor empowering but is rather a bargain with the system.

24. My MPhil dissertation 'Social Context of Girls' Education in Malabar Region (1900–1950)' in 1998 discusses in detail the social sector developments including education and the background factors. See also Tharakan (1984).

25. Kabir (2003) as cited from File no. 90 of 1932, L.G.B, Kerala State Archives, Thiruvananthapuram.

26. Research on hookworm, yaws, yellow fever, malaria, filaria and plague were of priority and matched the foundation's interest in the southern US. Before it reached Thiruvithamkoor at the request of the government, the foundation had already extended its activities to India. It was instrumental in founding the India School of Hygiene and Health in Calcutta. The Madras Presidency had witnessed a campaign on hookworms from 1919. A public health survey was carried out at the request of the Mysore government in 1927.

27. Only 19 deliveries were attended by qualified midwives in the year when the unit started, but after eight years almost 38 per cent of the births in the area were attended to by trained midwives.

28. Mary Poonen Lukose (1886–1976) was the first woman to attend B.A. classes and get a degree from the Maharaja's College, Thiruvananthapuram. She was the first Malayali woman to become a medical doctor. She became the Durbar Physician in 1924. She was born in an elite Christian family which was close to the power centre of Thiruvithamkoor. Her family was also influenced by European Christian practices due to its proximity with missionaries visiting from Europe. Her grandfather worked as an agent of the Church Missionary Society and her father, Dr E. Poonen, used to preach for the English missionaries. Her example is used by Jeffrey to

illustrate how women from well-to-do families chose to do courses in medicine rather than nursing, thereby highlighting the relative status of both professions in the hierarchy.

29. Abraham quotes from a publication in 1986 by Sr Candida Kandathil, *Indian Province*, privately published by the Sisters of the Holy Cross.

30. Census of India, as cited in Jeffrey (1992: 194).

31. A landmark Supreme Court verdict permitted Christian women in Kerala their rightful claim to their parents' property in 1986. It was on a petition by Mary Roy after a 30-year relentless campaign and struggle against Christian inheritance law that this was granted by the Court. There were many attempts to pass ordinances to restore the earlier position by the powerful lobby of Syrian Christian men, with the silent but strong support of the Church. This showed to a great extent the common interests shared by the patriarchs of the patrilineal families and the religious authorities.

32. Tarawad was the matrilineal institution that included the extended family, which in turn included the blood relatives, household and landholdings that had been inherited through the female lineage.

33. See the link made by Barrie Morrison (1997: 61–87) between migration and education as strategies for upward mobility by farmers in Kerala villages.

34. Nursing education, in fact, has never been free because nurses pay for their training by working in the hospitals attached to the nursing schools. This labour is not valued, not paid, and is seen as part of the training that the nurses receive.

35. It is often forgotten, even by nurses, that as trainees they compensate this by carrying out the duties of staff nurses in the hospitals. The argument of free training only makes the labour of these women invisible. Therefore, some nurses believe that the new system of capitation fees and increased tuition fees in nursing, especially in private hospitals, will in due course help raise the status of nursing.

2

Status of Nursing

The Sword of Damocles?

❧

Any discussion on nursing as a profession leads to an exploration of its status, job and migration opportunities, and its suitability for women as work. Status of the profession, of late, is discussed very much in connection with job opportunities, migration and the transformations in migration patterns. This marks a considerable shift from discussions based solely on factors of culture and purity-pollution which have dominated the concern with status in the Indian context. This is not to undercut the influence of these factors on the low status of nursing in India (Mohan 1985). Also important is the role of the Indian state. The state appears always—directly and indirectly—in the discourse on status of nursing, most often due to the paucity of its intervention in the health sector reforms.

In their efforts to develop a modern health care system, the state apparatus and agencies, nevertheless, attempted some measures. And the focus has been on the shortage of qualified manpower in all areas of clinical work including nursing. This was along the earlier patterns and policies that had given a direction to the sector at its nascent stage. In effect, this led to policies that made no clear distinction between different professionals like nurses (except medical doctors) and the paramedical workforce in medical care. And even when nursing was the focus of certain committees like the High Power Committee on Nursing, 1990, and Working Group on Nursing Education and Manpower, 1991, their reports remain largely neglected. An analysis of the historical development of nursing in the previous chapter has shown the stepmotherly treatment of the nursing profession which does not figure prominently in the recommendations of committees set up to formulate policies in comparison to the other significant one in patient care, namely, the medical profession. It is another matter that policies recommended in other fields also rarely translated into effective measures.

Some of the policies in the field of nursing were aimed to professionalise and standardise it in order to raise its status. University programmes created with this end in mind did produce a few nurse leaders; however, this did not have many positive effects on the status of staff nurses. In fact, this is believed to have widened the gap among various categories of nurses. One of the concerns that plagues nurse leaders in the current scenario in India is the amplified disparity between the faculty members and those in the clinical area.

This chapter looks at the historical evolution of status in contemporary discourses and its manifestation in everyday life, with special emphasis on the way nurses in this study perceive and experience it. Indian nursing is a profession on the margins (Nair and Healey 2006) that has been claiming independent status within the hospital hierarchy. Status issues are all-pervasive and part of the discourse on nursing across the world. For example, an analysis of nursing history and debates shows that nursing heroes were never part of the national history and, in the case of the UK, even prominent nurses who revolutionised the system were either not heeded easily in their own time like Nightingale or forgotten like Mary Seacole. The case is similar in country-specific studies—on France by Kergoat (1992) and South Africa by Marks (1994). As these examples reveal, status issues are neither peculiar nor specific to Indian society, though the interplay of caste and other ideologies of hierarchy, including gender in the Indian context, are difficult to unravel. Moreover, the colonial legacy has significantly contributed to the direction Indian nursing has taken.

Status Issues in India and Kerala: A Brief History

It is important to link contemporary concerns of status among nursing professionals in India with the historical analysis of status issues to understand and emphasise the elements of continuity. All the nurses in our study, to different degrees, spoke about anxieties related to their status. Gender, class ideology and practices of hierarchy, like caste, have contributed to the highly problematised status of the nursing profession. The colonial legacy and history of Indian nursing have simultaneously contributed to the professionalisation and the disquiet among nurses on the status of Indian nursing. Writings on the nursing profession in India reveal an uninterrupted orientation towards status issues from the past, as also the contemporary period. The first nurses' association in India, the Association of Nursing Superintendents or ANS[1], which was founded at Lucknow in 1905, stated that its primary aim was the professionalisation of nursing in India. 'Upholding in every way the dignity and honour of the Nursing profession' is stated to be a pre-requisite for which every nurse in the country must contribute her share. And this situation has not changed as could be seen in the discussions in the national seminar on Indian nursing after a century.[2] This seminar witnessed status issues being raised in every discussion in each session in some form or the other.

Yet the concept of status is too smooth to grasp; it eludes definition. This difficulty is exacerbated by the lack of a clear understanding of the term. Status has been understood differently by different disciplines, often seen by sociologists as intimately related to, but not necessarily indistinguishable from, class (Grusky 1994: 15–20). In the literature, status has often been seen to revolve around the ascription of honour (ibid.: 19–20). Evidently, status is informed by one's assets, occupational position and the ensuing societal appreciation. Writings on status in the sociological literature in India are mainly on customary status in the community and caste groups including that of ritual status and the standing of occupational groups.

The most significant factor in the understanding of nurses' experience of status seems to be the element of 'honour' or public recognition, apart from their service conditions. Nurses have pursued professional status, but the necessary degree of recognition of it by others is debatable. Although by definition nurses are skilled professionals who have mastered a specialised body of knowledge, in reality many of them have a knotty sense of their actual position in society. Clearly, many of them experience status not as a complete denial of respect for their profession but as a complex set of everyday experiences and, therefore, think about it ambivalently. This is inflated by the hierarchies within the profession in terms of the skills they acquire: a degree, a diploma or a certificate. Nevertheless, outside the profession the image of a nurse is a stereotype: the unskilled, morally suspect woman doing work similar to that of servants, subservient to everyone, including the patient and everyone else in the hospital.

Vagueness of 'status' creates difficulties in articulation even for the nurses though they are conscious of their professional identity. References to status in this case are often in comparison to other professions and people, as imagined by the nurses themselves. Nurses in this study experienced their status in relational terms, especially, as we might anticipate, with doctors, given the close proximity of their working lives in the institutional context of hospitals.

Sexual harassment at the workplace from colleagues, patients and workers, especially those on contract, is an expression of the unfavourable attitude that society shows towards women in public places. Sexual harassment has been an inescapable experience for many nurses and is attempted not only by superiors and doctors, but also by ward boys, relatives of patients and other workers in the hospitals.[3] Nurses on night shifts are particularly vulnerable to abuse and suspicion. The assumed deviance of being seen in a public space at night and their 'unusual' role as breadwinners is not easily accepted by society. Working with strangers, including male patients, leads to questions regarding the morality of nurses. This is also reported as the main reason for the very low participation of Muslim and high-caste Hindu women.[4]

As we discussed in the first chapter, the meagre material available on nursing in Kerala suggests that Christian missions' efforts in institutionalising modern nursing in Kerala (for example, Aravamudan 1975: 263–70) included recruiting women from underprivileged backgrounds. Nurses were identified as low-class workers from poor families and this added to the already defined low status of nursing. Stipends were offered to students, initially to attract more of them to nursing. This, along with the fact that they did not have to pay either for their studies or a job and that an income was assured at the end of the training, are described as the incentives for girls from poor families to enter nursing. The need for a job seems to have outweighed their concern for the potential damage to their reputation. Girls from landless poor families with minimum education looked upon nursing as a strategy to escape poverty.[5] Even recent studies on nurses reveal the class characteristics of nurse aspirants. For example, S. George's study on US emigrant nurses portrays nursing as an alternative to something else that should have been but could not be achieved due to the poor economic conditions of the family. '(T)heir families were not able to afford the expense (to go to medical school and so) nursing became a substitute' (2000: 150).

Low-class destitute women doubling up as nurses to escape poverty was identified as the most important reason for the low status of nursing and nurses even during its early days by pioneers like Hilda Lazarus, who therefore recommended that nurses from 'good and respectable' families must join the profession (Lazarus 1945: 11). Forbes (2005a: 94) reports that the National Council of Women in India, which took several progressive steps towards the betterment of women workers' lives like opening crèches and maternity benefits, demanded that the government make efforts to let more 'refined girls' enter nursing.[6] They recognised the poor service conditions of nurses as a preventive mechanism for 'respectable ladies'. It was also necessary to differentiate the modern nurse from the traditional midwife whose low-caste status also brought in questions of pollution for the profession's standing. The discourse on midwives of the new system as scientifically trained and therefore different from the dirty midwives of the earlier era helped create a space for women from higher castes and classes to enter nursing[7] (Malhotra 2003), but the suspicion of the women's status seemed to persist.

Nursing and Christianity has always had such a deep-rooted relationship that everyone in the profession was considered to be Christian due to its colonial and missionary connections. Christian missions in Kerala and the neighbouring states, especially Tamil Nadu, took an interest in developing a modern nursing profession in the image of their countries of origin. Christian converts were initially recruited for nursing. In Kerala, which has a substantial Christian population (19 per cent of the state population), there was an explicit understanding of nursing as a Christian profession and nurses as Christians. Many non-Christian nurses felt that nursing as a profession carried many characteristics from the Christian religion, like its professed attitude of compassion for the sick and elderly.

It is reported that there is subtle religious pressure on Christian nurses from Kerala when it comes to issues like abortion and that Catholic nurses take care not to go against the tenets of their religion. 'The church discourages women from working in hospitals that conduct abortions because the deed is against the tenets of the religion. The Fifth Commandment, which talks against killing, is for every Christian, including the nurses. We tell them not to become partners in killing and abortion is a killing', says Father Zacharia, Director of Jesus Nurses Fraternity which has 4,000 members.[8]

Nonetheless, we have also seen that though ideologies and practices of caste are important in the status of nursing, the first batch of nurses recruited by the Swiss sisters from the indigenous population were Hindus (Aravamudan 1975: 268). Pettachis in Kerala and dais in north India were primarily birth attendants and are equally indigenous. The former co-existed with the comparatively good hospital system and nurses in Kerala. Dais continue to be active, especially in remote areas, even when modern hospitals have been established, with their duties confined to the post-natal care of mothers and infants after deliveries in the hospitals, considered specialised tasks in themselves.

To the population outside Kerala, women who migrate to work as nurses in the hospitals of their cities are from Kerala and are Christians. Kerala, Christianity and nursing are seen as one and the same! However, much like their Hindu sisters, girls from affluent and powerful Christian families entered the medical care profession as doctors (Jeffrey 1992). That is, not all Christians joined nursing, and it is this complex interplay between religion, caste ideals and class which acted as determinants in Christian girls' decision to join nursing. Among Hindus and Muslims as well, class remained the most important factor in their choice of profession, though practices of gender seclusion made their public participation much more difficult than that of Christians of the same class.

Jeffrey's work on politics, women and well-being in the state of Kerala describes the life of Mary Punnen Lukose, the first woman medical doctor in Kerala. This illustration reveals a great deal about the widely prevailing class and status consciousness at the beginning of the 20th century among Malayalis, who treated nurses with utter contempt and suspicion, while patronisingly giving space to elite women in the medical profession towards the attainment of women's equality.

Thus, the modern Malayali who suffers from a chronically infectious patriarchal mindset, parodies a poem by a famous Malayali poet in praise of the spring that is in full bloom and has given the garden a new adorable look:

> *Aaruvanguminnaru vangumee*
> *aaramathin romancham*

The above stanza means: 'who will enjoy/buy the pride (masterpiece) of this garden?' is parodied as:

> *Aaru kettu minna ru kettu-*
> *mee nursin kazhutthil*

'who will tie *mangalsutr* on a nurse' neck?' This overly moral tone towards the sanction of nurses and their lifestyle is reflected in everything that appears in the media, including films. Numerous Malayalam films show the 'left behind' husband of a migrant nurse; the husband is portrayed as the victim of his wife's 'insatiable greed', while the wife is immoral and unresponsive towards the emotional needs of her family, that is, her husband and children. This trend of portraying nurses in a prejudiced fashion is also seen in Hindi cinema where the overt show of skin by nurses during duty hours is an idea fostered by directors and producers to ensure viewership. Only a furious agitation by nurses over the portrayal of nurses in the movie *Dil ka Doctor* led to some discussion on this issue in the mid-1990s[9] in the national capital.

'There is no Prestige in the Nursing Profession': Status in Nurses' Minds

The low status of their profession is manifested in the everyday experiences of nurses. This experience also sometimes is in association with the wide-ranging forms of expectations of stringent conformity to tradition from women of all groups. Working in both public and private sector hospitals as nursing professionals who are expected to look after sick persons, they do encounter low status in their everyday lives and that is a unanimous opinion regardless of their age and work situation. While nurses in the public sector admittedly are better off with a regular job, leave benefits and salary as per government rules, they are plagued by a very pitiable nurse-patient ratio and other poor service conditions. A constant irritant in their professional lives is the hierarchy in the hospitals that they feel negates their role in patient care. And this aspect is common with the private sector nurses who feel aggrieved by the lack of regularisation and standardisation of their sector. Ad hoc nature of their appointment and terms of work often leave their status in the hospital temporary without any right to leave benefits and stipulated wages. All this instability makes their sense of status even worse. The sample of the study was drawn mainly from hospitals in the private sector, 125 of the nurses were working in private hospitals of small, medium and large segments that mirror the organisation of hospitals in the health sector of Delhi. As pointed out, at the outset, 123 of the total of 150 nurses in the sample are below the age of 30, and these young nurses feel strongly about their low status and think of individual plans of escaping or avoiding it. The remainder were 30 years old and above, with the oldest being 51 years old.[10] Their articulation of their status differed, the younger nurses stressing on professional experiences as manifestations of low status and the older ones giving more importance to their personal lives, which, in their opinion, had given enough evidence to their low status.

The latter also emphasised the better state of nursing in the present as compared to earlier days. However, this indicated that there were differences in their experiences of status. Nurses in the age group 35 years and above (13 in total in the sample), with at least 10 years of experience, talked of their experiences 'before things became better', when the status of nursing was particularly problematic. On the other hand, the younger ones spoke more about what they had heard and their own practical strategies. There were shared feelings regarding the difficulty in getting marriages arranged for them. As in the case of Annamma Vijayan, they describe the entire process as 'humiliating' and how they are resigned to it: 'One proves one's innocence over a period of time to everyone who suspects the character of a nurse.' Thus, the onus is largely perceived to rest on the individual nurse. And the core of the self-criticism is constituted by issues of sexual morality and violation of the moral code of society by nurses.

At the same time, everyone whom I have met during my research believes that 'things are better now', that is, after 50 years of nursing in India. In the sample, 123 nurses less than 30 years old believe in migration as the only solution though everyone is not equally articulate about the status problem. Monetary improvement and exposure to technologically advanced hospitals in the Persian Gulf and in western countries are professed to be the panacea for their tribulations. Better service conditions and life chances due to migration opportunities to countries like the US and Europe are said to have improved the status of many nurses from Kerala. Many see status anxiety as inevitably linked to India, especially its culture, and claim that 'things would not be the same once they cross the seas'.

This optimistic view in Delhi is not corroborated by evidence elsewhere. In a recent study of immigrant Keralite nurses in the US (George 2005), there was an observed difference in societal standing between nurses' families and others'. There were many occasions when nurses' families, including their husbands and sons, have not been given the same treatment as others. For example, the trouble about marriage seems to persist even 'across the seas'. The marriage prospects of the children of nurses have been adversely affected by the condescending high-status families that consider nurses' status as low. Interestingly, in a context where everyone has made a fortune in 'El Dorado', the fact that nurses earn better salaries than many semi-skilled and non-professional migrants—especially men— actually works against them. Money matters less in comparison to hierarchies based on social and economic status back in the village. *Kudumba mahima*[11] of the ancestral family, including the position of at least two generations of ancestors, becomes important.

The moral status of nurses as a group is questioned even in an otherwise liberating milieu like the US (ibid.: 150). Questioning women's morality when they step outside the domestic sphere seems usual in rural patrifocal communities. Eugenia Georges' (1992) study on women and work in the Dominican Republic has a comparable situation. The late marriages of nurses, especially among the earlier generations, seem to have made them more vulnerable to questions about their moral and sexual 'purity', which are of utmost importance in the patriarchal society they live in.

Nurses in the study are well aware of the discourse around the moral character of nurses. Rani, for example, feels sorry for herself and other nurses who are 'good', because they have become victims to the 'acts of gossipmongers' and the bad name that nurses carry as a group. At the same time, she thinks that 'there must be a fire if there is smoke' (literal translation from Malayalam which is equivalent to the idiom 'there is no smoke without fire').

> ... I have heard so many times people talking about nurses as bad women...who are loose... but I know that I am not like that and I also know that my friends are not like that...I feel very sorry that people look at us like that... But you know...it is not completely untrue...there are girls who deserve that name and they make everyone stink ...get everyone a bad name...They really have no discipline and move around with boys who are said to be cousins...Everyone knows that they are no cousins... If you tell them not to do it, they stop talking to you...As a result men (Malayali) literally chase you thinking that "Oh! she is a nurse...(if I pursue her) she will come with me'...really.

It is clear that nurses too have started internalising the expectations and stereotyping. And what one realises is that these stereotypes have a life of their own. They float around, give you company and harass you when you are most vulnerable. Sometimes, stereotypes pass unnoticed, even by those who are being stereotyped. However, as stated above, nurses are aware of the stereotyping of the group and respond in diverse ways. Many are apologetic of the fact that there is a generalisation about every nurse and that they cannot help but feel bad about it, rather than question it. Some become defensive and project the 'noble' image of Florence Nightingale, denying themselves the right to assert themselves. This is very confusing and adds to the ambivalence of nurses as a group in dealing with issues in nursing. This also makes visible the divergent views nurses hold on the issue.

Mention of the word 'status' brought tears to the eyes of two respondents. In their mid-30s, both stood out as highly ambitious and very discontented at the time of the interviews. All the same, they said that their unsatisfactory professional positions are intertwined with their family finances and situation. For both of them their disappointment was not only the result of their lack of opportunities in their career; they were also dejected by the career graphs of their husbands. In fact, one of them, Sindhu, said 'there was no career' as far as her husband was concerned and 'so there was no question of a graph!' By taking up nursing they had expected something better than the deal they ended up within their family situation. They link their own status with the family situation, like the occupation and education of their husbands, and try to gauge what others think of their status, especially those with whom they interact on an everyday basis.

Case Study 1

Name: Sindhu
Age: 34
Caste: Nair
Religion: Hindu
Marital status: Married
Children: Two girls.
Husband: A computer programmer in a private firm in Safdarjung Enclave, New Delhi.
Self: Permanent staff nurse in government-owned Delhi hospital.[12]
Residence: Two-bedroom accommodation provided by the hospital within the same compound. Comfortable even for a large family in Delhi by her own admission. She also has a maid from Kerala to help with the housework and children.

I was asked to meet Sindhu for the interview at noon at her home. I was warmly welcomed by the maid who was talkative, looked overworked and tired. Since she was very well dressed and talked extensively on the family's life and Sindhu's routine, I took her to be her sister. She explained that Sindhu was late because her 'moped' had gone for servicing. I was told that she drives to her coaching class for the International English Language Testing System (IELTS) nursing examination. So I returned to the house at around 3 pm and was welcomed by an eager Sindhu who profusely apologised for not meeting me earlier. She was quite eloquent in her discussion on nursing and nurses. We developed an easy rapport, which was uncommon, as many nurses viewed me with suspicion. I learnt that she had been a very good student and obtaining high marks in the Kerala high school board examination, which is considered a deciding factor in a student's career plans.

> ...I wanted to be a doctor. I sat for the entrance test... But could not make it. I was reluctant to spend my time just preparing for the test though that was the trend at that time. I joined B.Sc. (Zoology) in a college at Ernakulam, thinking that I would try the medical examination again. But I had lost touch with the objective type of questions that formed the important portion of the medical entrance test. Again I could not qualify. All right, I thought. If I cannot be a doctor, I can be a nurse... A nurse is next in line in the hierarchy in the hospital system and in the treatment of patients... My father was a school teacher and could not really guide me but was ready to support me in whatever I decided to do...

Sindhu managed to gain admission in the nursing course in Delhi's Sir Ganga Ram Hospital by responding to newspaper advertisements. She worked there for more than six years before becoming a staff nurse in a Delhi government hospital. The test to enter the public nursing service is considered tough. She encountered her first experience on issues of status in Ganga Ram Hospital.

> I and another Malayali nurse were washing a male patient...in the ICU (Intensive Care Unit).... We were taking care of him as sincerely and normally as we always did.... We were about to leave when the next duty-nurse took over and a relative of the patient came in, very emotional and all that, giving us ₹100 each, saying, "Oh, you poor girls take this for taking care of our relative". We refused, saying that it was only our duty.... They became insistent: "... If not for money why would these girls come all the way from Kerala to work as nurses?" (addressing all those present there) "...You must be poor and not able to survive there"... We were in tears by the end of all that drama...

A second jolt to her understanding of nursing occurred when she got married. She was in love with her present husband who belonged to the same caste and village. He worked in a private firm in Delhi, and had no professional qualifications, earning less than she did. His parents disapproved strongly and wanted him to call off their relationship. But he stood his ground and his parents finally relented to 'bless the couple'. Her husband had to convince his parents that 'though Sindhu might be a nurse her character was good' and that it was no longer uncommon to find 'a nurse from good families' in Kerala. Sindhu is clear that it was the nature of her work as a nurse in a hospital that made her husband's parents so ill-disposed when they were otherwise quite nice and warm.

Sindhu would have been ready to put up with the low status if monetary and service conditions were better. It was not just a matter of her earnings but her husband's as well. He was earning ₹7,000 at the time of the interview, and she felt that he was not doing enough to improve his career prospects. In tears, she believed that it was because of her low status as a nurse that she had chosen someone with no career prospects. She would be 'restless' until she found a solution to her husband's 'lack of a career'.

This made her prepare for the qualifying examinations for nurses abroad (IELTS and Commission on Graduates of Foreign Nursing Schools or CGFNS) even though she had already received a job offer from Northern Ireland. What held her back was dissatisfaction over the amount offered as salary, and also Ireland's long history of conflict. She therefore applied elsewhere in the UK hoping to get a better deal.

Sindhu had no reservations about resigning from a permanent job, which she described as a good situation, and eventually left for Ireland. Making plans for the entire family's emigration, her husband left his job and the family anxiously hoped to join Sindhu later. At the time, he was about to leave Delhi for Kerala by the month end. I heard from a common acquaintance that Sindhu had sent enough money from Northern Ireland to buy a 'Scorpio' in Kerala, which was now plying as a taxi in her village. Thus, Sindhu had joined the flock of 'successful Kerala migrants'.

Case Study 2

Name: Parvathy
Age: 36
Caste: Ezhava
Religion: Hindu
Marital status: Married
Children: Two girls.

Husband: Is from the Yadava caste in Uttar Pradesh (UP) and works as a laboratory technician in a nursing home in Pusa Road, Delhi.

Self: Staff nurse in a private hospital in Model Town, north Delhi.

Residence: Rented accommodation in north-west Delhi. Travels by bus between work and home.

Parvathy brought up the class politics of the status of nurses immediately when we started discussing her experiences of status as a nurse. Her concern is not so much about doctors but about the general population's and patients' attitude towards women who come to work in Delhi as nurses.

> They [the Hindi-speaking locals in Delhi] consider us to be poor girls who have no means of survival back home [...] They look upon us in a bad way, but as we stay only with Malayalis, it does not matter that much. But I must admit that they are not all alike. It is those uneducated who are not used to see women going outside and work [...] The worst attitudes are those of rich patients without any education. They think that because they pay us, we are like their slaves.

Parvathy described her natal family situation at home in Kerala as abysmally poor at the time of her nursing studies, but it was not always that way. They were quite well-to-do when she was very young but her father became terminally ill and his business had to be handed over to his brother. Her mother was unemployed and in no position to help financially, and with three daughters. Parvathy had to travel quite far to reach her nursing school. She did not want to be a nurse and broke down at this point in her narration. She was not very clear what she wanted to become professionally or whether she wanted to work at all; therefore, her circumstances brought her to this 'considerably unsatisfactory situation for a woman'.

> I did not want to study nursing...There was no choice for me... Even my admission in the nursing course came about through a recommendation from someone who knew my father... He (father's friend) took pity on us. It was difficult for me to go for classes everyday from Kuttanad...I had no other options at the time but I also think that I could have got 'something better'....

My sister was in Delhi too. She is a nurse and married to a Malayali. But I married a North Indian…. Yes, it was a 'love marriage'… I had to decide all that on my own… [She smiled for a second and then turned very unfriendly. I reassured her that it was all right to stop if she felt uncomfortable; she ignored me and continued.]… I and my husband were working in the same hospital in Pusa Road and that is how we met. After I took leave for my first baby, I decided to start working here in Model Town because there was a break of five years …and joined this hospital.

Status issues were central to all the nurses I met. I discovered repeatedly that they were at the core of the protests that erupted around incidents that occurred in relation to their identity and work, and the discourses surrounding nursing. In fact, one important and most vital difference between the discourse within the profession and outside it has to do with the way status is dissected. In academic circles, status is generally seen as a 'complex' issue that is difficult to tackle and cannot be translated into words. But nurses disagree and comprehend status in terms of countable, tangible experiences with narrations that fill it with flesh and blood.

Status is derived from their experiences with their superiors (mainly doctors, and then administrators), patients, the general public, and subordinate staff in the hospitals. Nurses compared themselves to other professionals like teachers and doctors. The latter are the main reference group, which, they believe, are the main contributors like them in medical care. Their proximity to doctors also leads to the constant anxiety regarding their status vis-à-vis the doctors. Schoolteachers, according to the nurses, shared some similarities with their conditions, given that school teaching is also a woman-dominated profession. Second, like nursing, it is a profession that is viewed as appropriate for women. Some felt that teaching was better for women because teachers got two-months' paid vacation every year when they could be with their family.

Nurses have also viewed their status through definitions of professionalism and modernity. Invariably, the low status of nursing is explained as the consequence of the indigenisation that nursing was put through in India. The use of western uniforms and the English language (to help rid them of their inferiority complex) as the medium of communication became solutions offered for their low status. This argument sees individual Indian nurses as being responsible for the betterment of their status through 'improvement' of their behaviour and image in both public and professional spaces. Here the collective sense of belonging to a profession is not acknowledged and organising under the nurses' association or union is seen as a waste of time.

Anusha, 23 years old, for example, believes:

...white frocks...are traditionally associated with the service aspect and nobility of nursing as a profession and are very dignified. I do not understand why some nurses want to wear saris. First of all...it is difficult to manage. Second in the eyes of the patients, white frocks and the cap give an impression of power...It shows that nurses are professionals like doctors...And if you behave like slaves or servants, people will take you to be just that. Why do you put your head down when you walk across the room where all the patients and relatives and doctors are watching you? Come on... we cannot blame others for treating us badly when we ourselves do not believe that what we are doing is good.... As a nurse you are above the patients whom you are nursing. Show them that... then they will try to appreciate what you actually are. You will get what you are asking for. First of all, nurses have to believe that they are powerful and are in charge of the floor where they are working... then doctors will give them respect...

Mridula, another young nurse aged 24, who is her room-mate, nods fiercely in agreement. It is not just an impression held by these young nurses. In the public mind too the white frock is a sign of professionalism, albeit to a lesser degree. For example, the *Times of India*, in a report on Muslim nurses, says: 'Their spotless white uniform makes them look distinguished'.[13] Minocha (1996: 154) also talks about the role the uniform plays in patients' interpretation of the hospital situation. In that context Minocha says that nurses' uniforms invoked comments from patients and gave them some clarity regarding the status of nurses within the hospital setting. Patients, Minocha observes, are clear about doctors, as also the work and status of other paramedics, but their understanding of nurses' role is negligible.

While, in general, nurses think that they do not get their due as far as their profession is concerned, there are voices like that of Annamma (47 years old) who think that there are worse status situations for a woman worker than that of nurses. She locates status issues beyond the confines of the workplace, within the wider society. She does think that there are status problems in nursing and claims to have experienced them herself but it is not as bad 'as nurses make it out to be'. Her decision to become a nurse came from the intimidating behaviour of her male boss in her secretarial job; it was not only sexual intimidation but also her lack of assertiveness in managing her work that led her to change fields. She finds nursing to be better because it is a 'more public' profession. We will see how Annamma was able to evolve a more nuanced position on the status of nursing.

Annamma Vijayan joined nursing school at the age of 23 or 24, at a time when girls usually finish their studies and begin working as staff nurses.

> ... I had to sit with girls seven or eight years younger than me... they were more carefree... So I can say that I did not enjoy the classes much... But it was not a big problem. I stayed with my elder sister and her husband in Delhi.... I decided to do nursing after my experiences in stenography.... I looked upon nursing as work, work which you can do with self-respect, not like a secretary who is almost like a wife... looking after everything about (one's) boss...

She came to Delhi because her elder sister who was a nurse in a Delhi hospital brought her to do a secretarial-cum-stenography course at the YWCA in Delhi. The financial state of the family in Kerala was poor and she needed a job. She worked as a stenographer in two companies for a period of four years, but found the close intimacy with her male boss menacing. She was not an assertive person who could refuse work she was ordered and, thus, could not manage her role as a secretary without feeling dishonoured. She was allowed to go home only when her boss left, which was sometimes very late.

> ...Being a secretary was more like being the boss's 'wife'...I had to know everything about him...where he went...when he was coming back...I could not leave the work until he left...I could

not go on leave when I wanted...It had to be when he was absent from Delhi...Even Sunday he would call to ask for details about his travel or his contract with some company or a meeting...The rest of the staff would pass comments if I went with him in the car for a meeting...They were curious if I spent a few hours with the boss in his room which had restricted access (to other employees)... And it was mandatory considering that I had to take dictation from him... I found it difficult... I also saw my sister's job... My elder sister with whom I stayed (has been) a staff nurse...

Annamma joined Kapur Memorial Hospital[14] at Pusa Road in the 1981–82 session, determined to change her job. She was not bound by a contract to work there after the course was over. In 1985, Annamma started working as a staff nurse in a private hospital for ₹1,200 per month and then went to Saudi Arabia for a year. She found the job in Saudi Arabia unsatisfactory, with low pay and poor administration. It was a private hospital, where the chief of the hospital, who spoke only in Arabic, practically treated all the nurses, Indian and Filipina, as slaves. She returned and worked in another hospital before joining Ram Manohar Lohia Hospital in Delhi. When she joined, the basic pay was ₹1,400 for a staff nurse like her.

While working in Ram Manohar Lohia Hospital, she met her present husband. Her husband is a Hindu, a B.Sc (incomplete), and a travel agent with Panikker's Travels. Though her family was not against the marriage, they wanted him to convert to Christianity. He insisted that he would remain Hindu and she could remain Christian; his family had problems because she was a nurse. Their image of a nurse was of a woman who was ready to compromise on her character. The fact that she stayed away from her parents to earn money gave them the idea that she had a 'loose character like other nurses'. Until their son was born, she did not meet his parents, though he went periodically to Kerala to visit them. Her son is now 17 and she has a daughter who is seven. She told me that she considers her profession to be meaningful since she now knows about medicines and their use, and is able to advise her old parents in Kerala and others, especially in situations requiring first-aid. Presently there are no problems in her marriage because she is a nurse. She goes to church for Christmas, but her husband does not like her going to church often. She took her son to church when he was young but now he does not go except once in two years or so. Her husband does not go to the temple nor conduct any puja or rituals at home. The only religious emblem is a picture of Mother Mary. She has a bible, which she reads once in a while.

Her personal experiences again demonstrate the prejudice and misunderstanding about nurses, especially the sexual morality of women who mingle with strangers in hospitals. That was the problem her mother-in-law had with her, apart from the fact that she is Christian. But she feels that over time, when people get to know a person, they look beyond such issues and see you as a person 'who is good'. The best way to achieve this is to be patient, be yourself and do your work. She feels that misunderstanding is the main problem with the nursing profession, whereas the job of a personal secretary has the potential of misconduct by the male boss who interacts with you behind closed doors. The nature of the job is such that a secretary has to divulge the details of her personal life and that puts her in a situation of intimacy, turning the boss into a family member. Her sister's working life, in comparison, was better. 'You are not in a closed room with only your boss to whom you have to report; as a nurse you are in a public space, in a hospital.' Responding to the question of female bosses, she smiles and says, 'That is now, no?... there were not any at that point.'

Sitting very near the office of the secretary of the Delhi Nurses' Union (DNU), she says that she does not believe much in the collective actions that the union takes up, though this is better than not having any. She thinks that one has to fight one's battles on one's own, as she did in the case of her in-laws who were not willing to treat her as a 'desirable' bride. It is only society that is prejudiced, while her workplace does not put her in a difficult situation.

Her distrust of the DNU was more of suspicion towards the office bearers who, she thought, were biased in favour of nurses from north India. In small matters like granting leave or changes in allocation of shifts, one of the superintendents who is part of the union leadership, according to her, supports nurses from Delhi, whereas for Malayali nurses like her there is no mentor. Still, she attends the meetings and goes for protests organised by the union as she does not want to act like and be seen as a blackleg.

Annamma's elder sister also brought their brother to Delhi. Here he studied for a certificate in a government-recognised industrial training institute and married a nurse who works in Escorts Hospital in Mathura Road, Delhi. This was similar to the anecdotes by Tamil friends about Malayali migration behaviour, albeit exaggeratedly: 'Once a Malayali migrates to a place, the whole village will follow in a year'. She says that most of nurses' migration to cities in India happens like that. One nurse brings in many others who are in need of a job.

Sexual Harassment as an Extreme Manifestation of Low Status

During one of my interviews in Ram Manohar Lohia Hospital, after the night shift, a nurse was waiting for Mrs Khurana, the general secretary of the DNU to arrive. She was waiting to complain about an electrician who had been called in to fix a problem in the ward at night. He had been drunk and in no position to work. What is more, he tried to flirt with the nurse. Repeated attempts to get him out of the ward failed and eventually the nurse had to call security. This took up a lot of time since the nurse could not leave the ward, the phones were not functioning and there was not enough staff. She was afraid the whole night and kept looking towards the door. This was a female patients' ward. The problem was exacerbated by the fact that the electrician was not an employee of the hospital, but came from an electrical firm that was contracted to do electrical work and repairs in the hospital. This casual relationship between workers and the hospital creates difficulty for the complainant, which I witnessed when the nurse tried to report the matter to the medical superintendent the next day. Often it is difficult to identify the person. During night shifts, nurses feel unsafe and have to be extra alert.

The Shanti Mukand rape case of 6 September 2003 was still fresh in the minds of the nurses. This case made nurses panic so much that many wondered whether police protection would be necessary for nurses to continue working at night. A home nurse,[15] 19 years of age, was taking care of a comatose patient in Shanti Mukand Hospital. On the night of 6 September she was raped by a ward boy and in order to make sure that she would not identify him later, he gouged out her eyes; as a result, she lost complete sight in one eye and partial sight in the other. The callousness of the hospital in dealing with the case led DNU, along with women's organisations, to fight it out in the streets. This led to wide public support for the girl who belongs to a very poor family that had migrated to Delhi from Kerala about eight years earlier. The case brought to light the vulnerability of women nurses on night duty. Their defencelessness is greater in hospitals that provide poor service conditions to women workers including nurses. This case opens up associated issues like the lack of proper training for nurses and the absence of a regulatory body to provide home nurses with a licence.

While the above may be sidelined as the case of a personal carer and not a nurse, the much-publicised rape of Aruna Shanbaug, a nurse in Mumbai's King Edward Memorial (KEM) Hospital, in 1973 is a case of brutality towards staff nurses on night duty. In that case, too, a ward boy first choked the nurse with a dog collar and then raped her. She became 'cortically blind', that is, 'her eyes can see but her brain does not register any image. She cannot speak, emote, use her limbs or control her muscles'.[16] When she was raped, she was 25 years old. Since then she has been lying on a bed in KEM Hospital as her family and fiancé abandoned her.[17]

In fact, issues of safety and security of nurses figured prominently in the first strike by nurses in Delhi in 1967. Though hospital administrators acknowledge the need to provide safe working conditions, they are often implemented negligently. Most often, hospital administrators discuss sexual harassment as something that has to be prevented because it would affect the reputation of the hospital and that the media would sensationalise it; the safety of the nurse is secondary. Lack of physical safety is part of the poor working conditions that nurses encounter and indicates the low status a working woman like a nurse holds in the minds of the co-workers.

Nurses' Collective Bargaining

As we have seen in the previous section, lack of 'honour and dignity' in nursing caused nurses much anxiety from an early period of the development of the profession. Overcoming this problem became the first motivation for their collectivisation efforts and a show of strength. However, this approach put the responsibility for their honour on the nurses. Some of the earliest solutions for better status for nurses remind one of the reform movements among the 'lower' castes in the early decades of the 20th century. The way to attain the higher status enjoyed by the reference group, that is, the higher castes, was to imitate their 'better' habits—their rituals and cleanliness, both personal and related to the surroundings, vegetarianism and so on. The parallel in nursing is that they were exhorted to appropriate certain behaviour of the elite women, even when during situations like train travel! The solution was professionalisation and it formed a part of the vision of the earliest nurses' associations. Interestingly, this has been the case for many nurses' collective coordination efforts in the world. For example, in France, status and professionalisation formed important aspects of the organisational discourse in the 1980s and even later, as pointed out by Kergoat et al. (1992).

In India, the ANS, which was a meeting point of European nursing superintendents, took up the leadership role in 1907 with the aim of seeking 'the help and co-operation of Nurses throughout the country'. The Annual Conference in Bombay in 1908 decided to establish the Trained Nurses' Association, which was launched in 1909. The two organisations shared the same officers until 1910 (Dhaulta 2001: 211). Members of the Trained Nurses Association (TNA) elected their own officers at the first TNA conference held at Banaras the same year. The ANS and TNA were amalgamated in 1922 to create the Trained Nurses' Association of India (TNAI). Subsequently, the Health Visitor League (1922), Midwives and Auxiliary Nurse-Midwives Association (1925) and Student Nurses Association (1929–30) were established, in that order, to act as a forum where 'nurses could meet and plan to achieve these ends' (TNAI 2000: 7-9).

Nevertheless, the fact that the original organisational leadership was created by nine European nurses holding administrative posts in hospitals gave the efforts the lasting impression of being elitist. This proved an important point of departure by the nurses who formed the national leadership of public sector nurses in the 1980s and 1990s. The persistent status issues in Indian nursing are seen as a failure of the policies and practices of the TNAI[18]. Later mobilisations of nurses too revolve around status issues; one difference is that they have shifted the onus of the blame for the low status to non-individual, structural and social factors. This happened at two levels: first, shifting the responsibility for low status from the being and activities of 'a' particular nurse to highlighting the problem for the professional group as a whole. Second, collective bargaining and nurses' leadership is effective in fighting the status issue. This has been possible by identifying the historical and inherited legacies of Indian nursing, thus starting the search for an indigenous identity for nursing in India.

Mrs Khurana, who has been active in mobilising and organising nurses, censures external factors for the state of affairs in Indian nursing. She recognises that the historical neglect of nursing as a profession has contributed to the present dynamics. Condemnation of nurses as morally susceptible and weak professionals by the state and even by traditional trade unionists, according to her, led to the creation of the separate nurses' unions in Delhi's public sector hospitals.[19] Gender emerges as a clear marker here. Unlike most other professions, nursing has had to fight not just the barricade of the establishment but the strong and yet sometimes semi-transparent prejudices towards its practitioners due to their gender. The history of the Delhi hospitals' strike in 1985 was the rallying point for nurses' collectivisation.[20] Hospitals workers in the Delhi region declared a strike, demanding improved service conditions and salary increases. Nurses were active participants in the strike, although they were not part of the leadership that led the strike. It was assumed that issues specific to nurses, for example, long working hours, would be part of the demands put forward. However, the nurses' issues took a backseat when the workers' unions had to limit the number of issues during negotiations with the government. There were two points in the seemingly logical and neutral stand the trade unions took[21]: first, in terms of priority nurses' issues were not as important as others'; second, it pointed to the absence of nurses at the forefront of the strike. And, in a roundabout way, it indicated to nurses that, being women, their problems always got secondary importance in any agenda. Unmistakably, nurses' collective bargaining power was being questioned here. Thus Mrs Khurana identifies two issues: the organising power of nurses as workers and the capability of women to bargain for their rights as workers.

This surely acted as an eye-opener. Unionisation and collective bargaining 'by nurses for nurses' was found to be the only path towards redressals of their grievances. It was proven beyond doubt that the existing bargaining strategies—if any existed at all—were not doing the nurses any good. As a prominent nurse leader who voiced her concerns over matters relating to nurses, Khurana realised that an individual nurse in India is not in a position to deal with the whole issue of the status of Indian nurses. A nurse in India is already too burdened with her work, poor nurse-to-patient ratio, and pathetic working conditions. Moreover, it is not her task. Collective demands and the sheer strength of a united nurses' front were the only means to achieve that end. The TNAI did not seem to have the competence or inclination to undertake this task and they appeared to be far removed from the reality of the average nurse's life in India. She points out that the DNU came into existence in 1995 after this realisation. The majority of nurses by that time were convinced that their demands were consistently and systematically ignored by the leaders of the hospital workers' unions despite the fact that nurses had thrown their weight behind them in all situations. Nurses felt that they needed their own forum to voice their concerns.

What becomes clear is that the general belief, though contested by Menon (1992), that women are ignorant, disinterested and passive about collective bargaining was found to be untrue in this case. Nurses were active in the collective bargaining but the traditional trade union seemed to have a very patriarchal inclination as argued by Menon (ibid.: 187–96). The tendency to make questions pertaining to class the supreme point thereby undermining the gender issues also contributed towards women workers' questions being relegated to the background. As a result, visibility of women and women-specific issues in the trade unions became a casualty. Just as in the case of the cashew workers' struggle in Travancore that Anna Lindberg (2001: 217–84) speaks of, the leaders who organised workers in many protests were often women.

Assembling nurses for a common cause still seems to be a huge dilemma. Group consciousness and creating awareness among nurses about the numerous hidden issues that affect them professionally is difficult to begin with, but then this problem is shared by traditional trade unionists too. Beyond this, the very modes of gender relations in Indian society have a complex effect on the organisation of working relations within an institution like a hospital. There are parallels in every country of nurses having organised themselves. Kergoat et al. (1992: 115–25), for example, considers that the nurses' movement in France in the 1980s tried to incorporate the lessons of the wider French women's movement; in other words, the identity of nurses as women played the most important part in the institution of a collective body. Interestingly, and pertinent to our discussion, she talks about the term *infirmes* and its meaning as 'weak' that forms the root of the term *infirmière* (nurses) in French. Similar to that are the gender role expectations of women nurses as wives and mothers—the double burden, in other words—that put them in a tight spot in terms of time and energy.

Pushpa Suresh[22], is a good example of the double burden. Three years after my first meeting with her, she was forced to leave her job because her husband insisted that she was failing in her role as homemaker, unable to look after him and their children after her hard day's work at the hospital. Hence, she quit her job. At the time, while working she earned ₹3,500 but paid ₹1,500 to an *ayah* to look after her two children while she was on the afternoon shift at the hospital. She used the rickshaw instead of walking to get home as soon as possible. In spite of these arrangements, Pushpa described to me the guilt she lived through in leaving her children for work and of perpetually apologising for that to her family. This example shows that even while working Pushpa felt she was primarily and solely responsible for childcare.

Pushpa's case is typical of the average nurse who is caught between shortages of financial resources and time on the one hand and the stiff schedule of her gender roles as mother and wife at home. There has been an enduring sexual division of labour which women's work and employment has not changed. Most women, like Pushpa, run home after their duty hours; during duty hours they have no time for any organisational activity or rest. This has been found to be a fundamental obstacle in the mobilisation of nurses. Husbands too question the need for the nurses to stay back for matters not directly related to their work. Grace, 30 years old, had to face an angry husband when she went for protests to show solidarity with contract nurses in the prominent government hospital in west Delhi where she works. These nurses who were her colleagues—many of them from Kerala—needed other nurses' support and Grace understood that well.

> ...All that did not work with Achayan (husband) ...He asked me: 'Do you go to office for pothujanam or for yourself? Just mind your own business or you are going to be in trouble...If your work is finished early come home straight and be here... There are enough things here for you to worry over. Do not take on extra work ...' I had nothing to say... He is right...These people will not be there if the hospital decided to take action against nurses who went on dharna... But in the ward it was difficult to say no when other nurses were going for dharna... So next day again after my duty I went...I had to... Do you understand...? I work with them and I cannot be unsympathetic to them...

Then, there are conclusions that appear to be subversive to the feminist agenda: 'One woman cannot see another in the eye. Look at any mother-in-law/daughter-in-law problems in families... it is one woman who does not allow another one to prosper and be happy...' says Annamma who is 47 years old.

This was also the case with the engineers in my doctoral dissertation whose husbands thought that it was a waste of time for their wives to stay back for work other than the job at hand.[23] And yet Mrs Khurana feels that women nurses do participate in work-related activities when asked to, and when there is an efficient leadership. But she hastens to add that the support of the family, especially that of the husband, is important for women to play a role in public life. She brings forth her own case and even introduces her husband to me as the 'model husband' who not only stood by his wife but encouraged her to organise nurses. Mr Khurana says

> ... I fully understand the issues of nurses... I think that they really need to come together to fight... So when she (Mrs Khurana) showed interest in mobilising them, I fully supported her... I said 'if you want to spend your time even on holidays to take care of the issues related to nurses, go ahead'... I took care of children when she had to go out (for union work)... It was not easy but being active in nurses' union did not make her a less devoted mother...

He gives a sympathetic yet outsider's perspective to the nurses' struggle and testifies that status issues are central to their fight. Neither Mrs Khurana nor any of the other leaders with whom I had a group discussion are Malayalis. And no Malayali has been in a leadership position of the DNU though all of them participate in get-togethers that are mainly to protest against issues related to work or to demand better working conditions. Ancy Biju (43 years old) works in a Delhi government hospital and has been witness to many incidents that warrant protest and has participated in protests too. Despite this she is still reluctant to admit that nurses have to be militant in their protest to drive home a just issue. She articulates, in contrast to the majority in my sample, that nurses' unions in their present form are ineffective because they are apolitical and even non-political. She feels that this is because nursing is a women's profession. Women find it difficult to take part in politics because that is not considered 'good'. The only way to make others listen to nurses' concerns is by affiliating with political parties, acting as pressure groups and vote banks, and lobbying for one's cause.

> This is a democracy...My husband always says that this is the problem with nurses' struggles for their rights... Everyone thinks, what will these women do? ... After Mrs Khurana came to the forefront, our voice has been heard... News that is 'not only bad' about nurses comes up in the newspapers...It is not just about rape and sexual harassment...Our daily needs at work also get some attention.

She tells me that her opinions are a reflection of her husband's. He is the personal secretary to a cabinet minister with the central government who represents a constituency in Kerala. She informs me that most of the time she listens to discussions on politics and lobbying at home and realises how important these issues are. The DNU leaders agree completely. However, women's leadership still lacks the impact that men can make, and not just because of their inexperience but because they work in a public life with masculine traditions. As I found in my doctoral thesis on engineers and their leadership, women do not engage in networking outside their offices for career purposes as much as men, mainly due to the absence of such opportunities in women's lives.[24]

On the surface, the issues taken up by the DNU seem super-ficial. For instance, under the leadership of Mrs Khurana and others the DNU has campaigned to change the uniforms of nurses—white dresses reaching the knees and white caps—in government hospitals to saris and *salwar-kameez*. Many, includ-ing nurses, thought the change was absurd, while others wondered what difference the change would make. Delving deeper into the matter, one can read this demand as part of the challenge that Indian nursing today poses to its older legacy which it wants to throw off to stand as an independent profession. Mrs Khurana and the rest of the leadership in the DNU, contrary to the opinion of some of the young nurses mentioned earlier, felt that the western uniform exposed their legs unnecessarily and this was ridiculed and looked down upon by patients, especially those from 'uneducated and rural backgrounds'. She asks: what is the point in having an alien dress which only reminds one of a colonial legacy when the social reality of the majority of Indians does not fit that? She says that when patients are lying down on the floors of hospitals in rows because there are not enough beds, especially in government hospitals, how comfortable is a nurse walking through them in short dresses?

As mentioned earlier, these questions of indigenisation can-not be seen in isolation from questions of an Indian identity that nursing in India is trying to outline for itself. This should be interpreted as (re)claiming an identity—as a home-grown, Indian profession that is no longer a colonial creation. These are symbols of a rebellion in Indian nursing in their efforts to shake off the shackles of a western model that was imposed from above. Parallel to this and not yet unrelated is the discourse of occupational boundaries and professional identity. Women doctors who do not have uniforms are strongly discontent with the attempt of nurses to defy the dress code and this is seen as a challenge of professional hierarchy symbolically represented by the dress code. Uniforms, universally, carry a symbolic value for professions that has been underestimated and understudied.[25] Moreover, as Timmons and East (2011: 12) discuss in the context of the UK's National Health Service (NHS) Trust hospitals, doctors play the role of the arbiter of status for other professional groups in health care due to historical reasons.

A turning point in the DNU came in the wake of the ZEE Cinema production of a Hindi film called *Dil ka doctor* (1995).[26] This supposedly romantic comedy stars the famous Bollywood actor Anupam Kher as a doctor who has several love affairs with patients or subordinates in the hospital. There were many clips of nurses in short, revealing dresses in the movie trailer and advertisements in Bollywood style. Some of those who protested at that time, who are now part of the DNU, revealed in a group discussion that the projected image of the nurses 'basically shows a hospital as a place where everyone falls in love, does what they want and does no serious work. This added fuel to the fire... to already existing suspicions about the character of women who work at night in hospitals...'.

They organised themselves, moved the Delhi High Court and finally the film was withdrawn from theatres.[27] Mrs Khurana, who was in the news, was quoted as saying: 'In our country no woman can say with a sense of pride that she is a nurse by profession'. Even though no central government notification came through accepting the demands of the nurses for a change of uniforms to saris and salwar-kameez, nurses in Delhi started doing so on their own.

> It is the colour not exactly the change in the dress that is the problem with the authorities. We do not want to wear white. It is very difficult to maintain the whiteness, which turns yellowish in a few months. What difference does it make if nurses wear another colour? For us this is more convenient...

Not everyone agreed with Mrs Khurana and the All India Government Nurses' Federation, the national-level union of the government nurses, on the above point. Doctors thought that nurses were blowing the issue out of proportion and being over-sensitive about the portrayal of nurses in *Dil ka Doctor*. '*Dil ka Doctor* after all was a comedy film. I did not understand why they made a big issue about it?' one doctor confided, pleading anonymity. He says that doctors too are portrayed badly in many situations but they do not protest 'at the drop of a hat'. The nurses' agitation was at that moment taken as a sign of a growing lack of dedication among them, he points out. He insists that patients find it difficult to differentiate between a lady doctor and a nurse, which, in his opinion, is detrimental to the interests of the patients. However, nurses have been at the receiving end of sexist jokes for very long. It is no secret that it is only nurses' uniforms and not those of doctors that become shorter and revealing in films. Moreover, as found in the study by Timmons and East (2011) it is the group with higher status that feels aggrieved by the removal of specific uniforms and the subsequent 'mistaken identity'. Nurses also say that, unlike doctors, they do not have opportunities for career growth. Doctors counter this by pointing to research in nursing and specialised programmes like cancer nursing and neurosurgery nursing as possible openings.

The collective action of nurses in Delhi has centred on the questions of status—protests against what they consider to be the unfair portrayals of nurses and efforts to change what they believe are its causes, such as physical appearance and deeper issues like improvement in work conditions. All these, in fact, are efforts to stake claim to an independent status for Indian nursing as a profession. It is significant that the TNAI, which is more in the nature of a professional association of nurses, and the latter-day mobilisation of nurses akin to a trade union, share these concerns and yet approach the issues from different angles. While the TNAI tried to take up the issue of low status and asked the nurses to change their image by adopting lifestyles that are more 'respectable', the DNU rejected this approach outright. While the former followed the line of petitioning as a means of demanding the authorities' intervention, the DNU looked for mass mobilisation to draw the attention of not just the government but that of the public as well. Here the differentiation between professionals and labour comes out as well.

The discourse on the status of nursing and nurses everywhere (including in India), included plans to induct women from 'good and respectable' families and has suggested this as a remedy. Both caste and class aspects are implicated in such notions of the 'good and respectable'. However, the limitations of these arguments have been seen in the context of India where 'respectable ladies' would not easily enter into any engagement with the poor and low castes.

Wages and Status: Problematising the Connection

Status issues of nurses and nursing are always discussed in relation to wages. It is assumed that there is a direct relation between status and wages. Low wages are seen as part of the low status of nursing. When wages increase, status is assumed to rise proportionately. Monetary improvement for an individual nurse and her family thus contributes to a better overall standing of the family in the community and enables upward mobility. That is the rationale of many nurses who look for job opportunities in rich and advanced countries. When one looks at gender role expectations in Kerala, girls are a liability. This sense of burden changes to a great extent with women finding their own dowry (George 2005: 42–45).

Rise in status due to an improvement in economic position, is limited and constrained. Thus, a nurse who has a visa to migrate to the Persian Gulf or who possesses a green card may get selected as a bride[28] but not by families who do not need such avenues. Though not in the same manner as the male migrants described by Osella and Osella (2000), who depend on financial resources back home, women nurses do attain a certain level of status enhancement 'from burdens to assets' in the context of the original community in Kerala (George 2005: 42). Notwithstanding the merit of George's argument concerning the applicability of traditional parameters of status in Kerala in the migrants' space elsewhere, it cannot be forgotten that the change in the financial status is partly due to the huge exchange rate advantage of the US dollar. In the American context of the migrants too, nursing is not a high-status job and, as a result, non-nurse migrants transfer the same criteria of assessing status within the migrant community, even when family status (*tarawad mahima*) in Kerala is discounted.

But socially and experientially, status is more than what one earns and the relation between the two is more nuanced and subtle than allowed. In a curious way, nurses' labour gets more stigmatised in the community as their wages appreciate. As a nurse starts earning more in her job, her labour becomes more unmentionable as it does not fit the new persona made possible by the improved class position. Before long, her work profile is pushed to the background and the theoretical knowledge takes over as the important aspect of their work in their work descriptions, thus bringing them close, though not equal, to the physicians in their roles in patient care.

George points out that nurses' work is seen as 'dirty' in India: 'few nurses once they graduated and obtained staff positions in hospitals had to clean up after patients' (ibid.: 65). 'Dirty' jobs like washing the patient's body or removing the bedpan are not part of nursing work when it improves in status. Many Indian nurses find that in western countries some higher-level nurses do not mind doing these 'menial' jobs. But in the context of India's structures of purity and pollution, such work is demeaning and stigmatised (Raghavachari 1990).

Nurses' ways of dealing with their low status came out at the practical level in interviews. Migration to rich countries was clearly one way, not just for the better money but also for the changed locale. They also sought to remove what they thought were the stigmatised aspects of their job. They perceive nursing as dirty, lowly and humble and hence lacking in 'prestige'.

> ...removing the dirt and waste of a person is part of the nursing job. That is close to the work domestic servants do... How can the patient view me with respect if I am doing these things [removing bedpan, giving a bath, changing the bedcover and making the bed and so on]. They never think that I have studied in a nursing school for three and a half years and that too in English medium if I am doing all these things...rather I am like an illiterate woman who is ready to do anything to make a living... (Anusha, 23 years).

This opinion was shared by the majority of the nurses and nurse leaders, and partly reflects the 'purity-pollution' ideologies prevalent in Indian society. Nevertheless, they perceive considerable improvement in the status of Indian nursing and attribute this to two tangible 'material' changes, mainly in the environment of the hospitals. Technological changes and the use of more advanced and technically superior equipment give patient care an aura that is more credibly professional. Operating these machines for patient care enhances their status among patients that, in turn, boosts their self-confidence. And the employment of ayahs and ward boys to do certain 'lowly' and monotonous tasks like making beds, changing dirty linen and removing bodily fluids have helped create the perception that nurses are skilled and as a result more important in the hospital hierarchy. Ayahs, *methranis* and ward boys are perceived as subordinates who have to listen to the nurses' orders.

Elimination of these 'contemptible' tasks probably only removes the self-doubt of these women about the low status of their work and, therefore, gives them greater confidence in dealing with patients and fellow workers. Nevertheless, there is something about public attitudes that makes the status issue very sensitive. Sindhu, for example, says that she took all the caring work associated with nursing as professional and yet others' attitudes brought her to tears. She regrets her decision to choose nursing for a living. Here, one has to tread carefully, differentiating the need for better service conditions from assenting to the claim that nursing work is demeaning. While it is certainly the case that bad service conditions in India must be addressed at the earliest, it is equally necessary to focus on the other sources of nurses' low professional image and self-esteem.

As pointed out before, nurses think of Europe and North America as the place of salvation where they get better treatment. Except for senior nurses who are in leadership positions, young nurses believe that 'Indian cultural practices' are solely responsible for this situation. However, Rosemary Fitzgerald (1997) points out that nursing in western countries remained a 'disorganized occupation, mainly taken up by untrained or at best, poorly trained working class women'. A consultant in Ganga Ram Hospital testifies that in American hospitals nurses are depicted in pornographic pictures, wearing white dresses and in compromising positions with doctors. And yet studies like that of George (2005) and nurses who worked for a period of time in the Gulf argue that despite doing 'direct nursing work' — the 'dirty' aspects mentioned above—nurses possess a strong professional identity abroad, willing to 'do everything' to save patients there. Some nurses attributed this to better technological equipment and other's perception of nurses as 'professionals and people with medical and theoretical knowledge'. In fact, most of the nurses from Kerala are reported to have come to Delhi to get exposure to the technologically superior environment. Thus, there is a hierarchy within India where urban centres are reputed to have a number of technologically superior hospitals. Shiela (39 years), for example, points out that 'once you work here you cannot go back and work in Kerala hospitals.... There are no facilities there...'.

Considering that Indian nurses in the West also have to do physical work which they consider lowly here, why is it that they are more content there? The difference lies in their image of themselves as achievers by migrating to the US and in how their work is explained to them. They are well informed as to 'why they do certain things' and 'how those are going to help the patients'. This helps change their perception of themselves as important in the hierarchy of the hospital and as contributing in concrete terms to saving the lives of the patients (ibid.: 2005). Moreover nurses' professional identity is positively crystallised in the case of the US.

Hierarchy within the Hospital Structure

It is important to drive home the point that in their own minds nurses attach a very high status to the medical profession as a whole and a low status to nursing as it is practised in India. The theoretical nuances of a physician's education are admired by them as being exceptionally important and some nurses claim 'more equality' with physicians on the basis of 'we also study theories'.[29] Anusha, for example, differentiates nursing from a lab technicians' course and says that 'they do just a six months' course and their knowledge increases with each case that they do in the lab... But we do have a substantial amount of theory to learn about human physiology, pathology and so on....'. (She cannot find a syllabus and gives me a list of the courses in their nursing classes.)

Sindhu sees herself as equally or more intelligent than many of the doctors she works with. It is on the basis of individual capacity and not in terms of the superiority of the nursing course to other courses that she feels victimised. Her claim is based on the fact that she attained a distinction (more than 80 per cent of marks) in her high school examination in Kerala; she wanted to be a doctor but could not make it and ended up as a nurse. Working in close contact with doctors she could see the difference and resented it. Her disappointment with herself for not making it through the MBBS entrance examination puts her in a state of self-censure as well.

Figure 2.1 gives the common, skeletal hierarchy within the institutional context of the hospitals. Nevertheless, each hospital has its own organisational culture and working hierarchy, which is a slight modification, depending on factors such as the nature of the management and financial position and strength of the hospital. Nurse assistants (who hold certificates in nursing) are supposed to assist staff nurses who generally hold diplomas in nursing and are not full nurses. However, in most hospitals, nursing students are used as assistants or even as staff nurses under the supervision of a senior nurse, thus making the function cost-effective. The staff nurses are directly under the nursing superintendent. The medical superintendent is the highest authority in the hierarchy. Senior physicians also have complete control over the nurses and nursing superintendent, which is a manifestation of the gendered realities.

Some nurses, but not all, articulate the piece-meal routine of patient care in the Indian hospital and health care system

FIGURE 2.1
Hospital Hierarchy of Physicians and Nurses

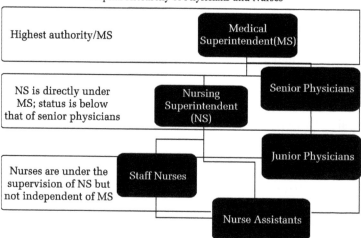

Source: Based on the researcher's observation of hierarchy within hospitals in India. Prepared by the author.

as one reason for the nurses' lack of respectability in the eyes of patients. Lack of holistic patient care and, as a result, the absence of coordination among doctors, dieticians, nurses and the rest of the hospital team lead to an overwhelming hierarchy within the hospital structure. This implies a system of overt discrimination against sections of the hospital staff that are lower in the hierarchy.

The relatively low position within the organisational structure, along with poor service conditions and a pitiable salary,[30] aggravate the status anxieties of nurses. The fact is that the medical hierarchy is a managerial hierarchy as well. 'It is a social construction and nurses, with other workers, and patients are active in producing it', points out Frances M. Gregor (1994: 219), illustrating the Canadian context. Aneeta Minocha (1996) through her study of Lady Hardinge Hospital in New Delhi says that patients make sense of the hospital hierarchy through the dynamics that they perceive in the ward where they are admitted and they actively participate in that hierarchy by interacting with each player. Patients' relationship with doctors and nurses is formed by the time spent by them in the ward and visibility of nurses vis-à-vis absence of doctors in the ward. In the case of her sample, most patients were ignorant of the role played by nurses and at the most were called *dawai denewali*[31] whereas thought doctors as powerful because of the latter's healing power. Doctors were seen as quite unlike them and language and physical appearance created a social distance between them and doctors.

We have already heard diverse views about the experiences and perceptions of status and how nurses have responded. There is unanimity that status is low but there is variation in how it affects each nurse, including in their perceptions and what each thinks of the effectiveness of their mode of response. Several of them feel that they are in a dead-end job, exacerbating the chasm between the other professionals they are in touch with daily, particularly the doctor who enjoys god-like status. Many perceive this as unjust.

There is also an unspoken rivalry between doctors and nurses, which doctors admit to and nurses occasionally articulate. According to one doctor who said he has been sensitive to the cause of nurses, doctors in general do think that 'nurses ask for much more than they deserve' in the hospital system. They clamour for no reason. Nurses on the other hand believe that doctors think of them as servants and of themselves as 'gods who alone can save the lives of patients'. Many doctors shout at them and treat them as subordinates and not as partners in the care of patients. The All India Government Nurses' Federation protests against the film *Dil ka Doctor* and subsequently against white dresses as uniforms in 1995 was one occasion when this contention became public. One doctor was reported to have said 'Nurses and doctors have to take an oath of dedication and responsibility towards the patients. So why make a business out of it?' There was also considerable opposition to the proposed changes[32] in nurses' uniforms from women doctors. Mrs Khurana alleged at that point that 'Even doctors feel insulted if patients mistake them for nurses'.

Nurses feel that they are seen as inferior and never as equal partners in patient care by the hospital administrators, doctors, other staff and patients. Instead, claim the nurses, they are crucial in saving the lives of critically ill/injured patients. Both Mrs Khurana and Mrs Manjulata have seen situations when critically injured patients were brought in at night and the duty nurses saved their lives with first aid and even went on to give further medication. In these cases the doctors were not available and the waiting time would have been decisive in the patients' lives. In situations when the doctor reaches late, instead of acknowledging the timely intervention of the nurses, they often scold them for their medication.

Thus, there seems to be a not-so-sympathetic relationship between doctors and nurses in Indian hospitals. This is not specific to Indian hospitals; Kergoat et al. (1992) illustrate the professional rivalry between doctors and nurses in France, where, for instance, nurses are the immediate subordinates of doctors and the case is similar in Canadian, British and South African hospitals. Gregor (1994: 224) explicitly mentions that the Canadian hospital system more or less excludes hospital staff other than physicians and the head nurse as part of the 'medical team' by failing to mention them. Mrs Sheila Seda, Secretary General of TNAI, mentions that omitting the names of nurses from reports on the teams that conducted 'successful events' like the first heart bypass surgery in India is very common.

Mrs Khurana too feels that hospital structures ensure that nurses are at the beck and call of doctors, because nurses come under the supervision of the medical superintendent.

T.K. Oommen, in his study of doctors and nurses within the framework of organisational role hierarchy, distinguishes between the two groups:

> ...the nurses have shorter periods of training, they do not usually generate knowledge, even when they apply knowledge to the decision as to what therapy is to be administered is made by the doctors, and they are supervised by administrative superiors or by full-fledged professionals (doctors) and invariably by both. These characteristics may lead to inertia, even erosion, of professionalism among nurses consequent upon their being employed in complex organisations, *viz.*, hospitals. In fact nurses invariably work in organisations whereas doctors work both in organisations and as independent practitioners. What we are suggesting, then, is that it is not the bureaucratisation of a profession *per se* which would eventuate in its deprofessionalisation but the degree of its professionalisation and the salient character of its work-milieu. (Oommen 1978: 12)

As Oommen points out, the occupational role hierarchy in the institutional context of a hospital puts nurses in a vulnerable position vis-à-vis their superiors. What is important is that the medical hierarchy is also a gender hierarchy. Like everywhere else, '(w)ithin medical hierarchy female-typed work is subordinated to male-typed work' (Gregor 1994: 223). While physicians' work is considered 'scientific', nurses' work is widely perceived as a manifestation of natural qualities that women possess and thus knowledge and skill and gender ideology go together in the hospital hierarchy.

Hierarchy within Nursing: Challenge to Sisterhood

Concepts of the profession and the professional bring forth images of independent practitioners and occupational organisations as Oommen (1978) points out. It was in line with this that, like elsewhere, the graduate nursing course was established. However, contrary to its intentions, the policy of bringing in a small number of handpicked graduate nurses to act as nurse leaders in India has brought in serious divisions within Indian nursing.[33] The first of these strategies to enhance the image of nursing as a profession soon created an uneasy rift between the university-educated degree holders (BSc Nursing) and the diploma nurses (GNM), trained in the hospitals of the conventional apprenticeship scheme.

At present the rivalry is not just between the graduate degree holders and diploma holders alone. Many under-trained nurses pose as staff nurses in nursing homes and small hospitals, without any evidence of training in nursing. We have a few of them in our sample and, despite their not having their diploma degrees (which is the minimum requirement for the post of staff nurse), I have included them in the sample in order to highlight the issues around them that include this hierarchy within nursing. Their presence in the health sector in Delhi poses serious challenges to quality health care and raises questions about the organised nature of Delhi's health sector. Private hospital managements are able to keep the nurses' wages low by employing under-qualified women.

The sample of my study in fact gives a sense of the lack of standardisation within the nursing profession. We have one person who completed her degree in nursing and joined a private hospital in Delhi in order to look for opportunities exclusively in the UK and the US. Two diploma holders have specialisations and both got their training from Batra Hospital, Delhi. There is one who did not complete her course due to family difficulties, including financial, six ANMs who have certificates from Kerala and two who never got a certificate though they claim to have been trained in an unrecognised institute in Kerala. Another girl who completed her lab technician course in Kerala was working as a staff nurse in one of the hospitals in south Delhi. One girl had no training and was working in a Special Economic Zone (SEZ) before she joined a small 15-bed hospital in north-west Delhi. The ANMs are examples of the underdogs in the profession who were remote from the paths of migration to any El Dorado. The vulnerability of the women who were joining the public and private hospitals under contract was also evident. Thus, there are several divisions and divergent service conditions among nurses in Delhi.

Media and the Status Issue

The media plays a significant role in enhancing and even creating the image of a profession and those who practise it. The role of the media and mass movements are critical areas to be analysed for the understanding of any group that advances its interests. And, amusingly, these are also the sensitive spots that are short of action in the case of groups that are struggling to attract attention from authorities and wider society. The lack of interest by the media itself is an indication of the low status of the profession of nursing. Absence of news is denial of space, and as critical media studies and poststructuralist standpoints state that there is a requirement to unveil the political and social construction of knowledge in the public sphere. 'Through the inclusion of some groups and exclusion of others, representations benefit dominant and positively represented groups and disadvantage marginalized and subordinated ones' (Douglas Kellner and Jeff Share 2005: 370). Often, successful lobbying and the subsequent achievements of the goals of the groups receive positive media coverage and this increases the involvement of group members. Fence sitters generally get involved at this juncture leading to mass mobilisation.

Search for news items and social science literature on nurses and nursing yielded very few results and not surprisingly so.[34] Under-representation has been an instrument used by the media that did not see nurses as potential partners in any sense. Mrs Khurana says that not under-representation but representation of nurses in bad light in society has been the types of news items that have appeared on nurses in the media, especially the print media. And this has done active harm to the image of the nurses. It is against this background that the author decided to concentrate on one incident that was covered well by the media.

Apart from print media, nurses feel that films too, especially Hindi movies that have global outreach, portray nurses as brazen women wearing skimpy clothing who 'play' with male doctors and patients rather than work. Advertisements and even items in newspapers on any topic related to hospitals provide a picture of a nurse in a short white dress even when it is irrelevant. All this apparently 'innocent' fun derives from and feeds into wider social prejudices. Mrs Khurana's query in the context of

Dil ka Doctor becomes pertinent here: 'Does comedy imply misrepresentation?'

When looked at against the backdrop of history of media and films in the representation of nurses, it becomes relevant to look at detail one of the incidents. The protest against the images of nurses in *Dil ka Doctor* was organised nation-wide by the All India Government Nurses' Federation. The *Times of India*[35] reported the following about the protest:

Nurses boycott uniform in protest against film

NEW DELHI, Oct. 4: Nurses across the country today did not wear their uniform in protest against what they called its vulgar and indecent depiction in the film Dil Ka Doctor.

Over 1,500 nurses took out a rally here denouncing the film, saying it had defamed the uniform and lowered the dignity of the noble profession.

A participant said the decision not to wear the uniform indefinitely would be taken today.

Secretary-general of the All-India government nurses federation G.K. Khurana, said the film had made a mockery of the profession and 'we will continue our fight to uphold its dignity.'

The above example is remembered as an important point in the depiction of nurses to society. Nurse leaders including Sujana Chakravarty and activists like Padma Prakash evaluate that a closer look at media reports since then indicates a slow change in the manner in which news about nurses is being reported. This is attributed to the belligerent unionism of the nurses. Yet there are nurses who would not agree that media representations are in anyway excessive. Mrs Khurana feels that the relentless engagement with the media has benefited the representation of nurses and nursing. The press was also under pressure due to the involvement of mass-based women's organisations like Janwadi Mahila Samiti (JMS)[36] after the rape in Shanti Mukand Hospital in east Delhi. The DNU and JMS, along with the National Federation of Indian Women (NFIW) and TNAI, organised a massive protest outside the Shanti Mukand Hospital on 16 September and kept a vigil till the time a verdict was passed. This case also shook the public by its gruesomeness. Though this was only one case of violent rape and attempt to murder, the media, including the CPI (M) party organs like People's Democracy, gave it substantial coverage.[37] The public outrage against the crime and support for the girl were largely created by and reflected in the media reportage.[38]

Unionisation and collective bargaining by the nurses has had some impact over the media, with some news highlighting their poor service conditions. More news on nurses' migration also appears, highlighting the poor quality of nursing in India as a result of these migrations. Also changes in the policy of host countries in the West that adversely affect potential migrants in countries like the UK have attracted considerable attention.

Though mass-based organisations like the All India Democratic Women's Association and JMS have always supported nurses' demands, their prior sympathy towards traditional trade unionists in hospitals makes it a difficult relationship. As discussed, despite nursing being a women-majority profession, academia or activists have showed very little interest in it. Does this incongruity exist because nurses' demands are largely perceived as workers' demands? In that process, have the ingrained prejudices and indifference to women as workers been ignored? The 'liminality' of the present health sector in Delhi that flouts the norms of the organised sectors of employment also confuses the understanding of nurses' working conditions and professional status.

Status anxiety—overtly and covertly—does mediate the responses of the nurses to the questions in their personal and professional lives. The image and status of nursing professionals are part of a universal discussion on nursing, similar to the cases in this study. For example, Daniele Senotier (1992: 23–55) says, in her analysis of the evolution of the profession in France over a century, that the history of the profession there can be divided into three phases. The first period (1878–1918) had a traditional, religious phase where differences between the profession and the vocation, duty and service emerged. Many new definitions sprang up along with the emergence of diverse sources of training. The second phase, till the 1960s, saw the growth of the nursing profession with more women coming in due to the two world wars and the spread of humanitarian ideas. Professional competence and the medical field also grew substantially. The third period that is currently on is said to have accelerated the specialisation of various cadres of nursing.

Across the world, modern nursing has had to fight certain collective notions that have worked against its growth as a profession; first and foremost, the notion that women are suitable for nursing because it comes 'naturally' to them. *Ni bonnes, ni nonnes, ni connes* (neither good, nor nuns, nor bitches) is one of the catchy slogans that nurses' organisations took up to protest against the exploitation and 'taken for grantedness' of nurses in France. Kergoat says in the context of the nurses' collectivism and unionisation that three factors have to be taken into account by any new effort to organise workers in a movement. First, maximum number of people should be part of the programme. Second, the group must look at existing associations, as also their relation to other groups. This leads to the third factor that nurses cannot ignore: the dynamics in the wider society while pushing for their rights. The South African nursing profession too has been plagued with many issues of a similar nature, complicated by the apartheid regime. Pursuit of professionalism through the tertiary education of nurses by shifting them from apprenticeship has not really helped the status of nursing (Marks 1994: 200).

One can see that the struggle to advance status and image and to improve service conditions is critically a feminist struggle. The fact that nursing is a women-dominated profession, at least numerically, is the most obvious but not the most significant reason for claiming the struggle to be feminist. Rather the issues that are dear to the nurses' movement are feminist in that they are up against an invisible frontier of gender and class pretensions. Some of the original nurses' associations in the earlier period of Indian nursing were attempting to question the elitism of other professions. Moreover, as elsewhere in the women's movement, the relationship between an articulation of the problem and raising a collective voice is central. Nurse leaders face strong customs and beliefs, on the one hand, and practices that have become normal in the public eye, on the other. Questioning them is offensive to public sensibilities and it is here that the media should play an important interventionist role.

Despite these parallels, the relationship between nursing, on the one hand, and feminism and the women's movement, on the other, seems to be an uneasy one. The word 'feminine', which is linked to nursing, is seen widely as diametrically opposed to the ideology of feminism. To be feminine and feminist seems to be a contradiction in terms in many minds, including some who call themselves feminists. This is because the popular sense of femininity at present is defined by patriarchy. This situation has its parallel elsewhere in the British context. In any case, like the women's movement in India in general, nurses have to learn several things from the West, which has walked a similar path; at the same time nursing in India must assert its originality, independence and identity and secure its own position within a globalising world.

The struggle of the movement of nurses to find their own identity in India is also a struggle against the past. In finding an indigenous uniform there are elements of post-colonial assertion by a group of women, who, apart from finding an identity of their own, are shaking up the overwhelming patrifocal dependence they experience just by being the appendages of their superior colleagues. Thus, the fight is at multiple levels. The agitation over uniforms by the DNU is not an attempt by conservative women to wear saris and salwar-kameez in their workplace. Nor is it an attempt to wear 'more trendy clothes in different colours' because white is not an attractive colour. (Some of the nursing professionals may, however, have a superstitious approach to white as it is the colour that widows wear.)

The case for better status is thus a complex one: At one level they have to get over the stereotyping of women as carers and show that they are professionals engaging in care-work and not women who are caring because it is natural for them to do so. At another level they have to reclaim their capacity to care because caring, in fact, goes beyond mechanical acts.

Notes

1. The ANS was later amalgamated with the Trained Nurses Association to become the Trained Nurses' Association of India. See the section on Collective Bargaining in this chapter for further discussion on this.

2. The national seminar, 'Indian Nursing in the New Era of Healthcare', was organised by the author on 2–3 December 2010 with the support of the Indian Council of Social Science Research (ICSSR), New Delhi.

3. In the first case, professional hierarchy primarily gives power to the harassers, whereas in the other cases the gender of the nurses makes them vulnerable to physical and verbal harassment.

4. A press report on nursing among Muslim women in the state of Maharashtra goes like this: 'Not a popular profession in the Muslim community. Conservative Muslim families don't encourage their daughters to take up a job which entails touching and tending to the opposite sex. It's extremely rare to encounter a Muslim nurse in this country. Even if families are willing to let their girls become nurses, clerics and friends would bemoan the decision' (Wajihuddin, Mohammed. 'When Nurses are Muslims', *Times of India*, http://articles.timesofindia.indiatimes.com/2006-12-17/india/27813741_1_nursing-school-muslim-girls-profession).

5. See Table 3.3 in Chapter 3 for the educational and occupational profile of nurses' parents in this study.

6. They also asked for compulsory registration of midwives, thus asking for standardisation.

7. Kerala women with modern education seemed to have entered this space with greater ease than elsewhere in India.

8. Wajihuddin, Mohammed. 'When Nurses are Muslims', *Times of India*, 2006, http://articles.timesofindia.indiatimes.com/2006-12-17/india/27813741_1_nursing-school-muslim-girls-profession

9. We discuss this later in the chapter but, at the outset, one must point out that nurses appear as consenting promiscuous women in hospital settings in the pornographic world where their agency in the act is overtly pointed out, as opined by some doctor friends who worked in the US. I am grateful to a consultant physician at Sir Ganga Ram Hospital for sharing his experiences and perceptions on this during our meetings.

10. As pointed out earlier the sampling technique depended on snowballing and availability of nurses for interviews and therefore does not really represent the opinions of the estimated 7,500 Malayali nurses in Delhi. However, the national seminar 'Indian Nursing in the New Era of Healthcare' validated the findings of this study as generic and as shared by nurses of all hues and colours.

11. *Kudumba mahima* can be roughly translated as 'family honour', which is beyond the material world though material success in the present or past is important and includes reputation, power and influence in the immediate village or community.

12. She works in a hospital in Northern Ireland now.
13. http://articles.timesofindia.indiatimes.com/2006-12-17/india/ 27813741_1_nursing-school-muslim-girls-profession. The report does not specify whether the uniform mentioned in the story is a frock.
14. This hospital, she told me, ceased to give training in nursing at some point in the 1990s.
15. She never completed her secondary school, which she was pursuing in Kerala due to the relocation, and was employed as a home nurse which did not make it mandatory for her to have a formal nursing education. This scenario is only possible because of the rather chaotic nature of the Indian health sector that has both formal and informal segments operating at the same time. This case is important because it is the case of a woman who was working, and being visible, at night. Lack of her formal affiliation with the workplace made her more vulnerable.
16. Kurup, S. 2006. 'Four Women India Forgot', *Times of India*, 7 May.
17. http://www.expresshealthcaremgmt.com/200701/market13. shtml
18. In fact, the TNAI has been forced to reconsider their 'pray and petition' policy, probably copied from our early national movement. The TNAI says that it 'did not believe in strikes and emphasised on peaceful negotiations' (Gulani 2001: 99). Though TNAI members refrained from striking for decades, some members joined the strikes and this led to a rethinking on the TNAI's part, eventually propelling them to give judicious support to strikes by nurses' associations.
19. Professionalisation never ceased to be on the agenda, though the responsibility for this process now swung from the shoulders of the individual nurse to structures of the health sector and hospitals.
20. The first-ever major strike in Delhi in 1967 marked the beginning of nurses' unionisation. Maharashtra, Kerala and Delhi started initiating associations of nurses. However, there was a divide among nurses regarding the 'spirit' of nursing and interests of patients while going on strike. However, over the next few decades, increasing numbers of nurses came forward to join strikes.
21. In this context, several papers in Milkman (1985) on the US women's labour history point out that the mobilisation of women has been especially effective when it has utilised organisational forms and techniques very different from those typically employed by men—forms that are rooted in women's own distinctive culture and life experiences.
22. Pushpa had undergone training as ANM but never got her certificate. In Delhi she worked in small nursing homes where her salary started at ₹1,000. When I first met her in 2005, she was paid the same. That

year she joined another nursing home where she was paid ₹2,000 and, in three years, she changed jobs in three small nursing homes. Since she had no certificate, it was not possible to apply to the big hospitals.

23. One chief engineer complained that her husband did not like it when people contacted her at home after duty hours. But as someone responsible for an area's distribution of electricity, people used to call her during emergency situations (Nair 2004).

24. Kiran Bedi's comments that lack of networking opportunities for women police officers like her are partly responsible for them being ignored in times of crucial promotions are applicable to women who are in top positions in all professions. My experiences with women engineers in leadership roles and senior positions point in the same direction. At the end of the day, a woman with the same capacity does not meet as many people who matter in social functions and therefore does not network as a man would in the same position.

25. Personal communication with Stephen Timmons, June 2011. Stephen Timmons is associate professor at the School of Nursing, Midwifery and Physiotherapy, University of Nottingham in the United Kingdom.

26. It was described as a funny but nonsensical romantic comedy about a middle-aged doctor. The film was directed by Avtar Bhogal Singh.

27. See http://www.cscsarchive.org/mediaArchive/medialaw. nsf/1105fec5535ec8ab6525698d00258968/1c65a18ee3460a 4d6525729c0025222b/$FILE/A0160155.pdf.

28. The nurses in this study reported that migration opportunities have a positive impact on their marriage prospects and status in wider society. As Marie Percot and I found, matrimonial adver-tisements in Malayalam newspapers ask for nurse brides with a green card and for those who passed the IELTS/CGFNS.

29. Recent nurses' strikes in Delhi hospitals took a more confrontational style which reflects the desperateness of the nurses' situation. They asked questions like 'what use are doctors when an emergency case is brought to the hospital? They are not even present in many cases.' 'Almost 70 per cent of patient care is done by nurses and why do they (doctors) claim primacy?'

30. The disparity in working conditions of nurses in private and public sector hospitals is overwhelming. At the time of this study, before the implementation of the Sixth Pay Commission recommenda-tions, the salary for a nurse was in the basic scale of ₹5,500 for

a fresher in a public sector hospital; the total salary of a nurse who completed General Nursing-Midwifery of three and a half years after her 10+2 was as low as mentioned here. The difference is even more glaring after the implementation of the Sixth Pay Commission recommendations in public sector hospitals. More about the working conditions can be found in the chapter on Delhi as a transit residence.

31. Literally, 'the one who gives medicine'. Aneeta says that nurses looked like doctors on one side and ayahs on the other. Nurses also exhibit the occasional tough attitude towards patients in order to make them obey hospital rules. Occasionally they also become friends with their patients and their personal care attendants. Thus nurses are put in a difficult situation as they manage the patients and the ward whereas doctors make an appearance once in the ward generally.

In another interesting discussion on the relationship between women doctors and nurses, some nurses claimed that women doctors treat them differently but some claim that women doctors take on the same medical ethos as male doctors. Pringle (1998: 187) quotes doctors saying that nurses in the context of England and Australia carry with them a certain understanding that doctors will treat them badly and they therefore report to work thinking what are we going to fight today with the doctors. Women doctors on the other hand felt that they were outsiders in the doctors-nurses relation because they did not have the authority that the maleness provided over the nurses nor sexual desirability of female nurses to male doctors. The same study also reports that women doctors face less sexual advances from other doctors and patients in comparison to nurses and their presence acts as a deterrent for nurses too.

32. To saris and salwar-kameez.

33. Probably this is not as unanticipated as is sometimes made out, since all professions create an elite group as part of its professionalisation and reinforce the divisions. Marks (1994: 13) analyses this process in the case of South African nursing where race, class and gender played dominant roles and says '...politics of nursing and professionalisation reinforced—and at times may have undermined—the divisions of a divided society'.

34. Similarly, Anju Vyas, librarian at Centre for Women's Development Studies (CWDS) made a presentation 'Researching Nurses and Nursing in India: Some Observations' in the national seminar 'Indian Nursing in the New Era of Healthcare' (see note 2). She reported quite in line with the author's experience that the reporting in newspapers with the keyword nursing also skewed towards

sensational events such as violence, protests, etc.

35. 5 October 1995.
36. JMS is an affiliate of the All India Democratic Women's Association.
37. See the coverage during the week of 21–28 September 2003.
38. At the same time, it was also alleged that the electronic media did sensationalise the rape and trivialised the issue of the safety of women at workplaces.

3

Choice of Nursing

A Life Strategy

❀

The women who participated in this research unambiguously convey the impression that for them nursing, as a professional choice, is part of a larger life plan. Nursing is a 'life strategy' rather than livelihood and stages of their personal lives are integrated into its various phases. Two aspects manifest themselves as important in their decision-making: (a) the family's role in a nurse's plans for the future (including their standard of living), and (b) improvements in the status of the individual nurse and her immediate kin. Whether or not the family is actively present in their decisions, it plays an important role in the way things turn out in their decision to take up nursing. Percot (2005), in her analysis of the Kerala nurses' migration to the Gulf countries, has also emphasised the significance of family in the decision-making processes of nurses.

I find that the role of the family in their lives cannot be articulated as a simple, individual family equation where the individual and family are monolithic entities, each acting for the well-being of the other. Sometimes, the absence of the (supportive) agency of family—the active inability of family to provide for and guide—in the lives of these women led to their taking up nursing. Access to information on nursing studies, work and migration opportunities and well-established female peer networks play important roles in their choices. Nonetheless, nursing is able to give these women something that other jobs have not. What might this be? How are they able to look at this as a life strategy rather than as a livelihood option?

An important point that emerges from discussions on the choice of nursing is that their future as nurses is intertwined with the processes and opportunities of migration. These perceptions are well grounded with their assessment of job opportunities and conditions of work in their immediate society in Kerala. This is followed by their assessment of prospects elsewhere. Thus, their choice of nursing and the decision to migrate are taken together. This chapter explores the complexities of their educational decision-making along with narrations of their experiences as nursing students. This recounting is retrospective and results in a flush of nostalgic sentimental memories, combined with accounts of the dreariness of it all. The period of their education was described as filled with drudgery; they were given all the menial work to do. Yet they cherish this period as the time of their awakening to personhood, of learning to take commands, and awaiting the moment when they would finally give them in return.

Understanding Educational Choices of Women Nurses

Education in the case of the nurses discussed here is described as training in a skill and is perceived as post-secondary school vocational education. This is validated by the classification of nursing as 'procedural knowledge' that includes apprenticeship. Though the GNM course involves three-and-a-half years training[1] after 10+2 years of school, it is seldom seen as higher education, which puts it at the bottom of the hierarchy of professions and occupations. Caring work is neither academic[2] nor is it theoretical, and the knowledge that comes with nurse training is not 'abstract' knowledge but rather manual and practical.

That is also why mainstream discourses on educational decision-making do not include discussions on nursing education. It slips between the discourse on higher education and vocational training courses, which in the Indian context is mainly technical training. The gendered nature of caring also gives way to this percolation. However, it is useful to look at the viewpoints of various sociologists, who use and modify mainstream theoretical frameworks and paradigms. Educational experiences are substantially influenced by the students' socioeconomic background. The education and occupation of parents and siblings form an integral part of the 'social class' of the respondents. This class dimension forms an important part of the discussions on nursing in the context of its perceived status in society and in hospitals, as we saw in the chapter on status.

Bernstein (1971), Bourdieu (1977) and others have been responsible for an extended and fascinating exploration into cultural capital and cultural deprivation. Feminist contributions to the understanding of educational choices and the experiences of women have enriched this discourse by adding the complex political connection between social expectations, assumptions and reality in women's education. The initial years focused on the increasing participation of women in terms of the relation between gender and equality in education. This was especially important in making education a tool for national development and making women partners in that process. Under-achievement and under-representation were subsequent emphases. Socialisation of the sex in the roles they play, and the consequent stereotyping of some subjects as suitable for 'feminine' roles, impacted women's educational decision-making adversely. This segregation of women into humanities and arts streams also received some attention. Links between the clustering of women in specific subjects and their occupational segregation later in life were pointed out. And yet nursing does not get any space in the debates and has been invisible except for sporadic mention in relation to other streams of education or as numbers among the growing skilled manpower of the nation.

Nevertheless, debates on perceptions of 'what is suitable for women' for their education are as applicable to nursing as to 'hard' subjects like engineering. Even among women who take up science subjects, there are patterns of segregation according to assumptions shaped by collective prejudice (Subrahmanyan 1998; Parikh and Sukhatme 1992). It is not a question of sex role socialisation alone but also of perceptions about what is practical and comfortable for women when they are supposed to be primarily preoccupied by their duties as wives and mothers. Most young women and their families take into account both monetary gains and marriageability (Mukhopadhyay and Seymour 1994). A profession like nursing, which is widely perceived as feminine, has been looked down on in the marriage market. Men from 'good families' have reportedly rejected nurse brides based on presuppositions of a corrupt sexual-moral character.

The gendering of subjects became the focus of attention of researchers like Jaiswal (1988) and Subrahmanyan (1998) who pointed out that some subjects are assumed to be masculine and others feminine, and boys and girls are expected to do better in 'their' respective subjects. Young children, right from the primary level of schooling, internalise this and begin to make choices accordingly. This is reinforced by the reward system of the schools and the mystification of science as subjects to be handled only by the hyper-intelligent, thus diminishing the value of other subjects (Jaiswal 1988: 8). It is argued that instead of seeking positive strategies to remedy the difficulties faced by girls in so-called 'male' crafts and subjects, girls are excused from performing well in these on the grounds that it is an unnecessary expectation for those who will spend their time in domestic tasks and child care.

Expectations for men and women are different 'from the moment they make a decision to train for a career. As graduate students, women are not expected to be as dedicated, ambitious, or serious about their studies as men. It is assumed that marriage and child-rearing will eventually interrupt their studies and certainly their career' (Kaufman 1984: 359). Moreover, women are described as emotional, irrational and therefore unsuitable for 'rational' subjects like science and engineering. In contrast, parents demand better performance from boys in these subjects. Various studies on women and science find that structural barriers like methodology and the content of science textbooks and the social structure of the lab work against women. In addition, definitions, images and the language of science are gendered (Carter and Kirkup 1990; Keller 1995: 27–31). This is where nursing fits in as a natural subject for women because of the nature of the work as personal care. Apart from 'gendered subjects', women have to face a 'gendered public place' in institutions of higher learning (Krishnaraj 1991; Subrahmanyan 1998:79–93). There are considerable social restrictions on the mobility and interaction of women students. Study tours, picnics and conferences that are organised help students through formal and informal learning and closer interaction often have only a few women students participating. This puts them in the backseat compared to boys who are able to make fuller use of such opportunities. Fear of sexual harassment, something that leads to extreme forms of social exclusion in India, also prevents women from attending these programmes and attaining parity with men (Subrahmanyan 1998: 129).

The existing literature shows that getting a degree in the subject of their choice does not come easily for women (Mukhopadhyay and Seymour 1994: 110; Subrahmanyan 1998: 79–93). Studies like that of Jaiswal (1988) argue that early socialisation practices coupled with sex-stereotypical education affect the entry, development and mobility of women in modern professions. However, this individualist view does not explain the decisions women make to pursue nursing after their secondary education. In this context, gender and class appear to be the most decisive factors in the educational decisions of women, taking into account the availability of livelihood options and converting these options into a life plan.

Karuna Chanana (2001) argues that the perceptions of women in terms of their primary role within the family makes women 'reluctant to describe themselves in career terms'; economic independence and autonomy take a backseat while marriage and housewifely duties take over as prime responsibilities. 'They do not want to drive single minded to top jobs' (ibid.: 356). These studies strengthen the need for a perspective linking education, work and family. General discussions and opinions on nurses tend to treat them as 'workers' rather than as professional women pursuing a career. But the interaction with the nurses during this study reveal that nursing is more than taking up a job and it is seen as the first step of a life plan aimed at social mobility, beyond the financial goals they set for themselves.

Educational Decision-making

In general, secondary education—schooling involving 10+2, and specifically examination results in the 10th grade—determines the direction that students' specialised training or post-secondary level education will take. In nursing, too, the two years of education after the 10th grade become important. GNM is the minimum level of training required for registering as a nurse and is the most common qualification among staff nurses in Indian hospitals. As mentioned earlier, this is a three-and-a-half year diploma after the 12th grade or a pre-degree.[3] Nursing schools in Kerala and public schools of nursing elsewhere admit only students who pass the 12th grade with science subjects, namely, physics, chemistry and biology. But there are private nursing schools (recognised by the nursing councils of the respective states) mainly in Tamil Nadu, Andhra Pradesh and Karnataka, and in some northern states like Uttar Pradesh, that admit students from any subject stream, including arts, humanities and commerce. They demand donations for admission into nursing programmes. This has led to allegations that the 'mushrooming' of nursing schools has not helped the nursing profession; rather, they lead to a dilution of the programme of study and a drop in the quality of nursing education which is anyway very precarious in small towns and rural areas.

The nurses in this study had all finished their pre-nursing studies in Kerala.[4] As shown in Table 3.1, Most of them (102 of 150) finished their two years education after matriculation in science courses whereas 42 in the sample completed their course in arts or commerce before pursuing their studies in nursing. When they found it difficult to get a place in Kerala's nursing schools, many chose to go to nursing schools in Andhra Pradesh, Karnataka or Tamil Nadu. My sample includes women who work as 'staff nurses' in small hospitals and nursing homes that are under-qualified for work in their present capacity. Among them, some are only qualified to be ANMs, since they only completed a year-and-a-half certificate course, while some merely attended a course in an unrecognised training centre for which they never even received an official certificate. Six in the sample either did not join 10+2 courses or did not complete them and they belong to this group. Table 3.2 shows the number of nurses in the sample according to the state in which they completed their nursing studies.

TABLE 3.1
Number of Nurses from Science and Non-Science
Background in Plus-two/Pre-degree Course

Age	Science	Arts/Commerce	Not completed	Total
22–30	80	40	5	125
31–51	22	2	1	25
Total	102	42	6	150

Source: Data collected from respondents through questionnaire and interview.

TABLE 3.2
Place of Training of Nurses in the Public and Private Hospitals in the Study

	Public	*Private*	*Total*
Delhi	16	37*	53
Kerala	3	36	39
Karnataka	2	14	16
Andhra Pradesh	1	18	19
Others	3	10	13
ANM	0	8**	8
No training	0	2***	2
Total	25	125	150

Notes: * One is a graduate in nursing from Delhi.
**Two did not get any certificates though were trained in ANM.
***One is trained as a lab technician.
Source: Data collected from respondents through questionnaire and interview

The maximum number of nurses in the sample received their training in Delhi, and the second largest segment came from Kerala's institutions. The training received in Delhi seems to have been advantageous for these nurses as they were able to gain employment in the public sector hospitals and private hospitals with a relatively good reputation in the city. However, most of the nurses who had just arrived in Delhi, fresh from the training schools, etc., were only able to gain employment in hospitals that were known to pay nurses poorly. It is here that network plays an important role, as we will see in the following chapter. All those who trained as GNMs from institutions in Kerala had a science background during their 10+2 period. The lack of a science background often forced the respondents to look for admission in institutions in Karnataka, Andhra Pradesh and Tamil Nadu. For those in the sample, donations to get admission in such places ranged from ₹ 10,000 to ₹ 40,000. Nevertheless, the nurses informed me that capitation fee was never asked for separately but is paid along with tuition and hostel fees. Though having completed a 10+ 2 course in science is a prerequisite for nursing in Kerala and in the government sector, nurses report that training in reputed institutions in Delhi and passing examinations like IELTS and CGFNS can overcome these 'minor' shortcomings.

Language ability (not just fluency, but also skill in answering tests) and the capacity to memorise short and objective type answers in the basics of anatomy, physiology and pathology help nurses get past the lack of science background for two years in their pre-degree or 10+2. That is why once those who are trained in the private hospitals of Karnataka, Tamil Nadu and Andhra Pradesh prefer to come to the urban centres and get exposure to technologically advanced hospitals. Shortage of nurses in places like Delhi is a boon for those who are looking for a foothold here. Thus, as much as a good academic record, hard work and networking are equally important to get past the individual limitations in terms of poor financial background and lack of training in A-grade institutions. Mostly the quality of the school and colleges is a matter of pride but according to nurses, 'it is the effort one puts in afterwards that ultimately counts'. One important difference, though, I observed is the difference in choice of destinations—to the Persian Gulf or to Europe or the US. Those who are confident of a good academic record think of the US and the European countries as destinations in their migratory plans while the Gulf remains a destination for those who are unable to pass IELTS and CGFNS and are not confident of doing so in future. But it is not exclusively these women who want to go to the Gulf; as mentioned elsewhere, the Gulf acts as a step towards the western countries as well. Again, those who want to come back and settle down in India look at the Gulf as the destination where they can earn good money with substantial savings. However, my sample had everyone unanimous in their ranking of the western nations as first in their preference and then the Gulf countries.

This is one of the reasons that nurses complain of lack of avenues for promotions, and this arises from an attitude towards nursing as a skill that is used on an everyday basis on patient care. Though not explicitly spelt out by Sindhu, the fact that she who thought herself as academically oriented and 'a good student' and someone who barely made it in matriculation do the same kind of work and are both called nurses seem to be a reason for her frustration and her need to 'make it big' elsewhere. The focal point here is the lack of professionalisation nurses experience in everyday work and, to some extent, the sense of permanence of work, salary and leave provisions according to the stipulated conditions give them some relief. Some hospitals in Delhi do not have many experienced nurses in their staff except for the supervisory posts; the remaining nursing work is done by fresh, migrant diploma holders (discussed in the next chapter). Diploma nurses in the sample who work in the private sector are those who faced some interruptions in their working life in India—a few of them had stopped working due to family commitments, while some had gone abroad to the Persian Gulf and came back to find jobs as staff nurse in the private sector easily. Personal interactions made it clear that they were not looking for any professional success at the present stages in their lives. Goals were defined in terms of family, financial security, and children's career and future.

Clearly, it is the quality and level of knowledge that nurses acquire that is being questioned here, and due to the shortage of nurses in hospitals not much attention is paid to the quality of education received by them. However, growing concern over the quality of nursing education is expressed by the leadership[5] and it is a fact that nursing occupies an ambivalent terrain between higher education and technical education, despite the fact that nurses undergo three years of engagement with textbooks in English, including practical training. Clearly, their education is under-rated considering the low percentage of women who continue their education after high school. John (2008: 57) presents the Gross Enrolment Ratios (GER)[6] in her analysis of 'gender gaps' in higher education as 10.57 for the female population that enrolled beyond high school. Understandably, we have to analyse nursing's concerns within the higher education literature. The existing literature on women's higher education demonstrates the interlinkages between gender, caste and class in women's educational choices and decision-making (Chanana 2001; Nair 2004). In the case of engineers[7] I found professional choices to be within the domain of family, where the heavy financial investment keeps matters within the power/control of parents. This is also true of nursing education in Kerala, though the total investment needed is much less than in medicine and engineering.

While the role of the family is central in choosing options in higher education and training, there is a difference in the responses of men and women engineers towards the question: 'Who took the decision that you would be an engineer?' In my dissertation, men did not hesitate to say that the decision was theirs, though their parents or neighbours had contributed, whereas almost all the women answered that it was the parent—the father in most cases—who decided their career. However, for both men and women the fact that they were making the most important career choice in their lives was undeniable. However, on going out of the domestic space into community places, the experience of the men differed from those of the women. While the men were confident in their decision and that 'it is their job', the women felt they had entered a strange place, though this did not involve any sense of incompetence as engineers on their part. Rather, the women's responses revealed how the importance they attributed to their own agency in decision-making was shrouded in anxiety and ambivalence.

In the case of the nurses, a larger number took the ultimate responsibility for the decision by voicing various logical arguments to support their choices. As discussed, the individual decision by each nurse was simultaneously a family strategy. The contradiction, if any, disappears with the explanation that the financial investment for the studies invariably came from the family, even when these women pay back the family or the institutions that offered them loans. And, social networks that contributed to their career moves were intertwined with the family in one way or another—even if sometimes only helping to maintain ties with their classmates and friends. Some older nurses take the entire responsibility for the decision-making, like Mariamma.[8] Smiling to me in a way to convey that this discussion was overtly amusing yet irrelevant to everyone else, she said:

> In those days nobody knew anything about studies... my parents were not educated (both are reported as illiterate)... They used to work as labourers (in small rubber plantations and paddy fields). Mother did not always work, though. Everyone was going to school and so we...five children...also went... everyone was going for nursing. You did not have to pay anything and they (hospital) gave you a stipend... not like what is happening now. Nowadays you have to pay lakhs of rupees for a nursing seat in Kerala... It was the neighbour who took me for admission. My parents did not even ask me what I did with myself...They could not be bothered when they were busy getting us food everyday. And after I joined, I asked my sister to join nursing as well and had the money to get her to Mumbai. She joined the nursing school of the hospital in which I was working... You might have heard the name JJ Hospital.[9]

For many older nurses and even the majority of younger nurses in my study the fact that nursing did not need much financial investment was an important factor in their decision-making. This is predictable given their socio-economic background. Now that more women, and even some men from the rich and middle classes, are taking up nursing, they prefer to do a degree (BSc) in nursing, failing which they opt for a diploma course (GNM), where most of the poorer women find themselves.

My respondents made frequent comparisons between physicians, teachers and nurses. They preferred teaching to nursing, given its respectability.[10] However, they cited several reasons why many did not become teachers. First, their marks were too low to get into a Teachers' Training Course. Second, nurses' training was seen as less strenuous though involving more hard work. Third, teachers in Kerala have to pay a 'donation' to get a job. As the brother of one respondent, Reena, pointed out, intervention by powerful people like politicians, caste and community leaders has become necessary to get a job in Kerala.

This comparison between teaching and nursing is an ongoing one, even in the minds of institution builders. For example, a news item[11] on the new trend of Muslim women entering nursing reports that it was school teaching that was previously considered ideal for women who needed economic support. 'We thought nursing would help empower women in a better way than teaching does', said Sayeeda Dadarkar, general secretary of the college run by the 75-year-old Anjuman Khairul Islam Charitable Trust which was now starting a nursing school.

Gender and Class in the Exercise of Their Options

The discussions on the nursing profession and its status emphasise nursing as an employment opportunity for women who have few other options. We have already traced this legacy, including how the first recruits were mainly destitute and needy women. Even decades after women entered nursing, the association of nursing with candidates from poorer class backgrounds continued. Nursing thus came to be understood as a low-paying career for the economically desperate. In the beginning, it was an occupation for a distinct social class—impoverished, formerly low-caste Hindu converts to Christianity. Later, it became associated with a distinct segment of Kerala society as, from about 1932, Malayali women with high-school education and a serious need for an income took up nursing (Jeffrey 1992: 193–95). Class status still remains a major reason for women to opt for nursing, as expressed below in the words of Bindu (age 26), a young nurse from Kerala.

> 'Being from a family which has just enough to survive, it is necessary to stand on one's feet and earn one's living... Doing any of those general courses like B.A. or B.Com does not help because you do not get a job in Kerala or elsewhere if you do not have political patronage. You also have to spend money for your studies. So I thought about nursing... The investment needed is affordable and if one is willing to migrate to other states one will surely get a job. There is no hospital in any part of the world where there is no Malayali nurse. As such Malayalis are everywhere in the world and so are Malayali nurses.'

Nursing is chosen as a career because the number of years spent studying and the investment required for the courses are relatively low. Three years of training in GNM after 10+2 ensures a job in Indian hospitals and possibly abroad. In the case of engineers, my earlier study, a job was important to raise the life standard of their families, whereas in the case of nurses a job is necessary to sustain their families. While it is said that the class background of new entrants into the nursing profession is slowly changing to include better-off families, I did not encounter this during my study. The women I met during my research were looking for a source of livelihood. The income they earned from nursing was going to decide their future economic standing and the direction of their lives.

Women in Kerala hear that a nursing diploma guarantees jobs in hospitals in states outside Kerala from relatives and friends who work there. The other factor is the economic position of their families. Most of the nurses in my sample come from families that are small landowners or labourers, where the father is the main or sole earner. As Table 3.3 shows, the majority described their fathers as farmers or small shopkeepers (94 out of 150 respondents). The fathers of 48 respondents were employed as

TABLE 3.3

Educational Qualifications and Occupations of Parents of 150 Nurse Respondents

Educational qualification	Mother (in numbers)	Father (in numbers)
Illiterate	1	1
Attended school/ Dropped out before class 10	40	37
Passed Class 10	77	84
Graduates	31	20
Post-graduates/professionals	1	8
Total	150	150

Occupations	Mother (in numbers)	Father (in numbers)
Landless labourer	1	6
Farmers (2-5 acres of land)	nil#	52
Clerks/Soldiers/School teachers	9	48
Self-employed other than farming	3	42
Professionals	1	2
Housewives	136	nil
Total	150	150

Notes: Many of the occupational categories are overlapping. For example, homeopathic physician who is classified as a professional is also self-employed.

Bias of the respondents in the classification of fathers alone as farmers while mothers reported as housewives even when they are involved in manning the family-owned small land-holding is to be taken into account. One mother was reported as agricultural labourer though not a farmer.

Source: Data collected from respondents through questionnaire and interview.

clerks or technicians in the government or private sectors or had retired from those jobs. In six cases, the father was a labourer. The mothers were invariably described as housewives, yet many of them contributed to the family by working as labourers or through small, informal poultry or dairy farms. Brothers and sisters were also employed as middle-level employees or as farmers or nurses, except in rare cases where the brothers were earning good incomes or pursuing vocations of their liking.

All the respondents specified 'job opportunity' as 'the single most important' reason for the choice of migration. 'We all know that there are no jobs in Kerala. Anyone who comes across us on the road has a BA or MA degree and is still looking for a job...' (Reena, 26 years).

Availability of nursing jobs in hospitals in India and abroad is the primary reason for nurses taking up this course. Studying nursing and taking it up as a profession were deliberate choices and not passive experiences, as the stereotype about nurses in Kerala would have it. Their trust in the by-now time-honoured tradition of nurses' migration for jobs to other states gave them the much-needed encouragement that they would not experience unemployment. If you are a nurse 'you can get a job in at least a nursing home in Kerala too…Salary may be low… sometimes they pay just ₹ 1,000…But still you will get something for your sustenance…'

One aspect that strongly emerges is that while a graduate in arts, humanities or pure science is seen to have no job possibilities, nurses acquire a skill that provides them with a livelihood. This is an important dimension of the status of nursing. Its vocational characteristics lend it immediate appeal, but at the same time devalue it. Those who are looking for a job find it attractive, whereas those who can 'afford to think' about status are in a dilemma over the class dimension. After eliminating various courses as being unsuitable, nursing becomes the job 'best suited' for needy women. Along with this is its suitability in relation to femininity and marriageability. A 27-year-old nurse, Babitha, from Kerala who works in a private hospital in Delhi says:

> Nursing is one of those professions where girls can perform well. A nurse has to be in touch with the pain and feelings of the patients. It is easy to get a job once you are trained as nurse because it is a field where Malayalis and women have established themselves.

Gendering the subject of nursing becomes the major explanation offered by women who chose this profession. Nursing is an example of how women get segregated within defined sectors of the labour market as an occupation which is seen to be an extension of women's traditional role. Women are said to make good nurses because they are 'naturally' caring, conscientious about details, have nimble hands and soft manners and are sufficiently submissive to take orders well.[12]

In the context of the 'masculine' branch of engineering, teachers find that girl students are often enthusiastic about taking up subjects like mechanical engineering but are discouraged by their parents who believe such subjects are not good for a girl's future; by this, they mean that the work profile of a mechanical engineer does not suit women's roles as wife and mother. Thus, in the case of engineers, women's options become constrained by social expectations. Less social independence and mobility of women make them opt for a job with fixed working hours (9 am to 5 pm, for example). Choosing electrical engineering was rationalised as an effort to get an office job which does not require travelling into the field. In the case of nurses, night shifts at the workplace were described as both an advantage and a disadvantage. While night shifts are taken to be obstacles to a comfortable family life, some nurses think that eight-hour shifts enable them to use their daytime effectively, for example, taking part in their children's school activities.

While nurses in the sample were unanimous in their opinion that nursing is suitable for women, they are ambivalent in their opinion on the clash between nurses' notions of ideal womanhood and the requirement for nurses to share a public space with strangers even at night. Women are subject to frequent and ubiquitous moral suspicion as a result of being nurses. Except the nurse leaders whom I met, no one in the sample made the link between the gender identity of nurses in wider society and the issue of harassment of which they are all aware and against. Widespread opinions have linked nurse work to prostitution due to their supposed deviance from 'ideal' womanhood (Nair and Healey 2006). Even among the missionaries who were pioneers in nursing education, it was perceived that nursing students and nurses were morally suspect. There are many veiled and some not-so-veiled references to the lurking dangers of prostitution in their writings on nursing and nurses even in the context of the UK. These have always been linked to the low status of women in Indian society, often also carrying the inhibitions of their own culture to India.

Mukhopadhyay and Seymour (1994) also discuss the role of traditional norms on gender roles prevailing in society. They identify the agency of the family in negotiating between traditional norms in society and modern education for girls. The role of the family, as we have already seen, is absolutely central in the choice of nursing as a profession. But it cannot be ignored that the role of the family could be 'forced' in retrospect. Female relatives and a network of friends provide the main support and inspiration, and were identified as 'significant others' by nurses. Women classmates and neighbours provide nurses with vital clues on affordable nursing schools at a distance from their homes. These female networks play the most important role in their decision-making. But nurses look forward to the support and approval of their families in all their decisions. And in some cases it is the pressure of this expectation that makes them retrospectively attribute to the family a strong role in making choices.

It is interesting to compare the case of engineers and nurses regarding social prestige and reputation. Engineers do not report any trouble in getting married due to their job per se, though some of them report late marriages because they had to wait for men with higher or equal qualifications and social status. While some families value a science and engineering degree, they recognise that arranging their daughter's marriage gets complicated because they will have to look for bridegrooms who have a better education and higher degrees for their highly educated daughters. Practices of hypergamy and the conventional belief that husbands should outrank their wives are widespread. 'Traditionally age, caste status and worldly knowledge tended to constitute such criteria whereas today educational status has become a major criterion of male authority and family rank' (ibid.: 14). Though educational decisions are taken ambivalently due to the stigma they face in the wider society, nurses do use nursing and the existing marriage system as strategies to their advantage. They marry men with higher degrees in general courses that may have little job value in the market but who are nonetheless more educated by conventional standards. If one examines the matrimonial sites of newspapers aiming at Malayalis, a bride with a visa to the US and Europe becomes the ticket for overcoming the loss of status associated with nursing. However, it remains a fraught strategy, carrying potential social and marriage risks. Casual conversations with Malayalis who are not nurses indicate that, among other factors, it is the ambivalent status of nursing in the marriage market that also keeps many from joining.

By comparison, although engineering is viewed as masculine and may not be compatible with the social image of the 'ideal woman', doing engineering[13] is socially prestigious due to the ascription of a higher-class position. 'Several expert consultants though professing support for women's entry into science and engineering admitted that they viewed their sons' mathematical competence as having significant family impact, requiring investment in a tutor; in contrast, their daughters' success was pleasant but relatively inconsequential' (Mukhopadhyay 1994: 109). This shows that investment in girls' engineering education is the result of a better class position to begin with. In the case of the engineers in my study, their class position allowed them to invest in girls' education, whereas for nurses nursing was the only professional course they could afford. As Subrahmanyan (1998) points out, in the case of girls' education, questions about the financial viability of a father supporting a daughter's education arise because gender roles within a family are well differentiated and only a son is expected to be a provider.

Nurses reported that in earlier days women in nursing used to remain unmarried because men from 'good families' were not ready to marry them. Also, nurses in military services could not get married according to the law. However, young nurses in the study say that new possibilities of emigration to rich countries have improved the demand for nurses in the marriage market. This is how they rationalise their life strategy and make their future plans, right at the point when they choose nursing education. Here is a typical life plan, versions of which were detailed to me by several respondents: after completing their education they would migrate to one of the cities of India, like Delhi, guided by the networks of friends and senior colleagues there. The individual nurse in question would then accumulate at least the two years' experience required to get a nursing job in one of the Gulf countries; during this period she would try to obtain high enough scores in the IELTS and CGFNS examinations to make her passage to Europe or the US. Experience in a super-speciality hospital adds to her curriculum vitae. The money earned at this time is the money she plans to use for the expenses to apply for a job abroad. While she is in the Gulf, she will get married and then, along with her husband, migrate to the US, which is the first preference, or to Europe, Australia or New Zealand. In case of failure, there is another path which, Shiny, for example, calls 'Plan-B'; this is a return to Kerala in case of pregnancy and then a renewal of the work contract in the Gulf after leaving the child behind with the mother or mother-in-law.

Thus many of the women I met in Delhi were in the middle of carrying forward plans that were hatched when they were nursing students.

Bindu, quoted earlier, decided to take up nursing to also facilitate her elder brother's desire to take up painting as a profession. She told me that she had taken over the responsibility of providing for the parents and the family as her brother, who was expected to be the provider, had not yet started earning enough to do that. She has one brother and two sisters and the family could only afford to invest in their brother. Even though she also paints well, she decided to confine this to her leisure time and work as a nurse. She said that the decision to take up nursing was solely hers because she wanted to be self-reliant and wants to help her parents monetarily. Her family had taken bank loans for her education, which she was repaying during the period of my interviews with her.

In the broad survey of the hospitals that I did initially, with the ultimate aim of selection of sample for interviews, I did not come across any Muslim nurse. This has to be clarified as I faced many questions about Muslim nurses. They do not generally migrate alone for work, unlike the Christian nurses, due to stricter adherence to practices of seclusion. Religious ideologies, gender practices and class factors combine to create a complex, adverse decision-making process for Muslim women. Understanding the complexities in this area helps us better understand the decisions of nurses. When Muslim girls become nurses often they do not disclose their profession to neighbours and relatives. Even mothers do not want them to be a nurse. Families allow them to take this 'radical career choice' under the condition that they would tend only to females.[14] Muslim girls who are undergoing training are from impoverished families. Nursing institutes mentioned in the above story faces immense pressure from the clerics. 'They quoted scriptures saying Islam lays emphasis on women's modesty. Undeterred, the college responds with an instance from the Prophet's times when Rufaida, one of his female companions nursed the injured during a battle'. Consensus in the community seems to be that the "scriptures do not stop women from becoming nurses as long as they do not flout some tenets".[15] The same report says that contact with patients and hospital paraphernalia is stigmatised in the north Indian population in general, and not just among Muslims.

The marriage market is prejudiced against nurses and that works as a disincentive. The dais in north Indian villages were from the Chamar caste and this association is seen as a blemish in a casteist society for women of other castes.

We have seen how class positions as well as the class aspirations of nurses in the sample played a vital role in their educational decisions. Traditional gender norms, economic compulsions and status seem to be at odds in the case of nurses. Aspirations of escape and some class mobility result in viewing education as the route to an individual's economic security and betterment of status. 'It often has a profound impact on the welfare of the entire natal family—its economic welfare, its ability to secure 'good' marriages for family members and its overall family status...Hence, educational decisions, like marriage decisions, are not left in the hands of individual students' (Mukhopadhyay 1994: 106).

Nursing Schools

The demand for nursing has increased since the inception of the allopathic hospital system and availability of jobs in hospitals. Some regions like Kerala had the highest demand for nursing courses, and schools of nursing in Kerala could not accommodate them. Visa and job opportunities opened up due to the development of the hospital system in India, the oil-rich Persian Gulf countries and the shortage of trained nurses in western countries. The criteria for selection and admission are particularly strict in Kerala and that led many nursing aspirants to look for schools elsewhere. Thus, a significant proportion of my respondents studied nursing outside Kerala. Experiences in the nursing schools were described on the whole as pleasant, though full of responsibilities. Student nurses are expected to do all the tedious work associated with sick patients during the period of their studies. According to some of them, this period was very stressful because any mistake in patient care is easily blamed on student nurses. Student nurses are condemned to hard work; their labour is seen as of no value and is taken for granted and not paid, as it is termed 'training'. In some schools, the training was difficult to endure, principally because of the behaviour of the doctors and senior staff nurses involving much shouting, etc. In fact, the cheap labour of nursing students acts as an impetus for many hospitals to start nursing schools. This, to a great extent, cancels the shortage of nurses in the hospitals, adding to the profits of the hospitals and influencing the notion of 'nursing work' as charity at best and free in most cases. This also sustains the resistance shown by the hospital management against improvements in salary structures and service conditions.

Nursing duties were described as difficult and the super-intendents as 'strict disciplinarians'. Their descriptions of their experiences in this regard remind one of the discourses on permissible conduct of nursing students during Florence Nightingale's periods in England. Bijitha who hails from a small town in eastern Kerala did her GNM course in a mission hospital.

> …I did my nursing in Cherthala in a Mission hospital… Sisters (nuns) were very strict…We could not go shopping… We had to buy things when we went home or some nuns would accompany us when a group went shopping…The only place allowed was the church on Sundays and someone had to come from my home for us to go home…it was only 70 kilometres…This nursing school is famous for its discipline…

According to the respondents, their parents consider the con-vents run by nuns as the next best option, besides themselves, for the safekeeping of their daughters. In Kerala, many parents prefer convent schools run by nuns due to their strict rules and discipline.

> It was hard for me to leave home early… It was especially difficult during exams and night shifts…I wanted to stay in the hostel. But my parents did not want me to be away…for two reasons. Being a girl, it was proper for me to stay at home and travel everyday. These days 'bad name' is very easily thrust upon girls and then it is difficult to remove that. And my parents had little money in their pockets… It was financially difficult even to pay my fees, buy clothes and give me money for bus travel everyday… So I did not insist. I could understand the problem. But it was impossible to travel during exams… I did stay with my friends with special permission from the wardens of the hostels… Sometimes they frowned but generally they agreed (to allow me stay over)…I was scared to request too often. I had to get a letter from my father

each time. Otherwise they just did not permit me to stay with my
friends... (Reeja Philip, 24 years)

The restrictions imposed by nursing school matrons are well
supported and often complemented by parents with a heavy
hand. Shijy, for example, remembers her school days as very
difficult to manage and talks about her father as a tyrant. She felt
that she breathed fresh air only when she left her home for Delhi.
And she rejoices in the freedom that the new space gives her. For
her, the limitations as a woman started at home and the toughest
frontier to cross was that of the 'patriarchal father figure'.

It is no wonder then that though women like Shijy talk
about these issues, most prefer to keep quiet. I believe that
P. Chatterjee's (1994b: 132) assertion in the context of undivided
Bengal, that 'the battle for the new idea of womanhood in the era
of nationalism was waged in the home', holds true even after the
nationalist ideology won over the colonialist British decades ago.

In the words of many women, patriarchal society's best manifestation was home and the nurse matrons. There is no contradiction in the strident binary of the domestic and public[16]
which is taught to them. And, in fact, the question of women has
been articulated within the domestic space and the domestic
space is where the woman is disciplined to adhere to the values
taught to her on her behaviour in public.

Those who studied outside the state of Kerala had no option
but to stay in hostels. Financial planning had to include the
expense of board and lodging.

> There was no problem in the hostel (in Andhra Pradesh)... Of
> course it was expensive in comparison to the option of staying
> at home but it wasn't that costly in comparison to the hostels in
> Kerala. We had to pay the hostel fees along with the tuition fees
> at the beginning of each year. Once that was done, we were not
> bothered for a year. We—me, my sister and parents—put aside
> the money in advance each year. I managed to finish my studies
> within the budget. Once or twice, I had to ask for more money...
> for my train journey to attend some function at home ... I had to
> make that extra trip and in another case I fell seriously ill and had
> to be home for care... My hospital was good enough but I wanted
> to be at home...near my mother...*Their (family members') care is
> better any day*[17] ... (Sheeja, 27 years)

Apart from these limitations, there could also have been difficult experiences involving misbehaviour towards nursing students who were rendered more vulnerable because they did not speak the local language and were under considerable financial stress. Such students could not think of leaving school without finishing the course, as they had no alternate opportunity awaiting them, not to mention the financial burden shouldered by the family that had invested in their education. Recent media reports have alleged cases of sexual harassment of migrant students in nursing schools in Andhra Pradesh even by male members of the school management.[18]

Yet, in retrospect, all nursing students think of their student lives in nursing schools as satisfying and lively with 'a lot of things happening during that period'. The spirit of camaraderie and sisterhood developed during these years is common to all students who stayed in the hostels. They made friends and developed the networks that later helped them find jobs. Those who described themselves as 'day-scholars'—who stayed at home and commuted to the school everyday—were reportedly less involved in group activities and were outwardly 'less happy' about this time of their lives. They had to leave home very early and catch buses to reach school on time. All of them had to stay in the hostels at some point, at least for short periods, or when they were allotted night shifts as part of their floor duties during the course.

As students, they were not only concerned about family finances and personal matters, they were making enquiries and investments for future jobs. Seniors who were about to leave the schools were important sources, as were classmates whose neighbours, elder sisters or cousins were employed in Delhi or other such cities in India. Thus, migration across states of India and abroad is part of the 'nursing strategy'. Here there are different kinds of planned movements—direct emigration to the UK, Europe or the Gulf (West Asia) for the few who could afford it. But for the majority a longer life of migration is expected to be part of their lives, before they can settle down with their families. Their typical thoughts on settling down include Kerala, a husband and two children as the basic ingredients of their future dream. Unmarried young nurses between 22 and 27 years in my study had these elements firmly in place when they thought about their future. Thus, nursing is a 'package' that contains a job, travel opportunities, some individual freedom, marriage and wedding plans including 'family planning'.

These discussions also suggest the importance of ethnicity and the location of girls in the decision-making on their education. Discussed in detail in the next chapter, networks among nurses in Delhi become important in the decision-making on nursing as well. A number of 'significant others' assume the role of helping hands in choosing the location of the nursing school. This is often based on their understanding of the ranking of nursing schools, their reputation and the expected expenditure. While in the case of the engineers of my doctoral study it was a mixed group of teachers, parents and neighbours, both men and women, who provided information, nurses primarily relied on women who already work as nurses. Advice and help received from parents was often negligible in the case of nurses. This also reflects the low educational background of most parents.

A comparison of nurses' and engineers' attitude towards their career brings out interesting dimensions in their career expectations. Nurses think that they 'meet with life directly' (that is, deal with matters of life and death), while engineers think of themselves as participants in national development. Engineers view themselves as tough professionals, whereas nurses perceive themselves as softer, more gentle and caring, as being able to be in touch with others' feelings, emotions and pain. At the same time, nursing is looked at as providing care that is 'less than professional' even by some nurses. The values nurses possess as individuals are undoubtedly influenced by their class status and gender, thus highlighting the interplay of class and gender in their decision-making.

Nursing Education: Issues of Status and Strategy

Ignorance about nursing education and training, even among relatives and professional associates, leads to a devaluation of the education they receive. Nursing education is not seen as education and training in the way that engineering is, for example, but is a 'low status trade' as pointed out by George (2005: 41).

Nelson (1996: 6) argues in the context of academic disciplines like economics that 'judgement of worthiness' of the subject is based on masculine norms. It is the same models that define nursing as low in the hierarchy of educational options. An important dimension of the devaluation of nursing is also the difficulty of quantifying the actual work involved apart from the menial work that is associated with nursing. For example, the 'kind and straightforward' communication that nurses are supposed to engage in with patients is not an easy category and is not measurable and comparable; nevertheless, it is an important part of their work. Discussion with nurses and social science researchers from different European countries also suggested that this is a universal problem.

This has been the case from the beginning of nursing history. Though religious missionary efforts in nursing brought in certain images of it as a noble profession, the fact that in the initial years, at least, those who took up nursing were those driven by economic necessity and by the unavailability or unaffordability of any thing better paid or better regarded has not been forgotten.

Even the missionaries who became involved were not free of prejudices towards the class from where early nursing recruits hailed. For instance, Hilda Lazarus[19] wrote:

> Those in charge of orphans were anxious about their future and decided thus: if a girl were pretty she was sure to get married, if good at passing examinations she was made a teacher; and if she possessed neither of the former she was sent to be trained as a nurse or midwife.20

How do nurses in my sample look at nursing? Do they look for a job or a livelihood? Respondents gave wide-ranging opinions on nursing as a profession and as a skill. It's first and foremost is a livelihood option but goes beyond that and assumes the role of a life plan because of the nature of engagement they have with it. Chanana's (2001) argument that differences in career involvement and professional commitment among working women vary due to differences in their compulsions and motivations will be an interesting point to deal with in depth. She says that the above differences arise from differences in their socio-economic status and the nature of occupations.

Perceptions towards their own work can differ:

> For instance, those who are in low-status and low-paid jobs, such as clerks, nurses and school teachers, are more likely to be working because of financial necessity... (Chanana 2001: 357)

Even when nurses look primarily for a job and a livelihood, as is evident in the study, their lifelong engagement with it in order to ensure a better standard of life for themselves and their family makes it different from being treated as just a job. A typical nurse in my study is focused on security and money that is very much the characteristics of a job-holder, she is also ready for risk-taking and learning and on the job training in order to improve her job prospects. The main target is economic and subsequent social mobility. I would argue here that the differentiation between a job and a career is not very tenable in the case of nurses just on the basis of the common characteristics.

This discussion suggests that class and gender norms and ideals decisively influence and inform nurses' educational choices. These choices bring in new options in terms of their prior class positions, but at the same time reinforce the traditional constraints of the gender division of labour. There are rising aspirations among parents and young women for a profession that ensures high social and economic status. Even in the case of nurses whose choices are seen mainly in terms of 'saving the family' from impoverishment and insolvency, these are accompanied by a reinforcement of traditional norms and gender relations which nurses play upon in order to gain their own rewards in the system. Evaluated according to how useful it would be to their future, the choices of nurses cannot be seen in terms of a simple 'preference'. Being a woman and a nurse are defined together. Social approval is also important.

Supposedly neutral educational institutions also promote gender stereotypes and actively shape girls' perceptions of their own roles and behaviour in wider society. 'Patrilocal' structures of family and ideology continue to play a major role in women's academic and professional choices. It is also found that some families send daughters only to local, lower-ranked institutions for higher studies rather than prestigious institutions in distant cities because the second option is socially risky for girls (Mukhopadhyay 1994: 112; Subrahmanyan 1998: 85).

The social and economic status of the parental family led to their decision to take up nursing. Concerns regarding the future of their families and their future roles in the families are strong influences in their decisions. Socialisation and understanding the social role of men and women, as also class compulsions, seem to persuade women towards certain educational decisions. Unrelenting alertness and hard work along with social networking provide the nurses, nevertheless, with the 'power to choose' from the options, however limited they are.

It is clear that nursing offers the best opportunity to those who are ready to migrate to other states and even outside India. There is a difference in the approach of older and younger nurses in Delhi towards nursing as a life strategy. Due to the increased opportunities for migration abroad, unlike older nurses, staying in Indian cities has not become the final step in migration. Cities like Delhi have become transit spots where their plans are operationalised at multiple levels. Also, 'saving for dowries' is postponed to a later stage and saving to pay entrance fees for examinations like IELTS and CGFNS has become the norm, as discussed in the next chapter.

Notes

1. Nursing courses are post-secondary programmes of BSc (four years) and GNM. ANMs, health visitors and health supervisors are nurses who can assist the registered nurses. Recent developments in nursing education show that more and more private institutions are incorporating BSc programmes in nursing into their curriculum where at one time this course was the exclusive domain of public sector colleges.

   Higher level courses include Diploma in Nursing Education and Administration (10 months), MSc (with clinical specialisations), MPhil (one year, full time and two years for part time), and PhD in Nursing.

2. Professionalisation of nursing attempted in India and elsewhere focuses on this distinction between theory and practice within nursing, leading to a sharp hierarchy within nursing.

3. Pre-degree is a two-year course after the Secondary School Leaving Certificate (10th grade) and before the student enters college for undergraduate courses. This course used to be conducted in colleges which were associated with universities. This was replaced by the 10+2 system in schools, in a phased manner, and the 10+2 is now the model that operates in most Indian states. The last batch of the pre-degree course in Kerala was in the year 2000.

4. Except for two nurses in the sample who lived their school years in north India because of the transferable nature of their fathers' jobs.
5. This was a major concern raised by experts in the Nursing Research Society of India (NRSI) and Centre for Women's Development Studies (CWDS) consultation held on 7 July 2011 on the proposed survey on the status of nurses as well.
6. She uses the data computed by Saraswati Raju (2007) from various rounds of the NSSO. Figures for the male population, urban women and rural women for 2004–5 stand at 14.42, 22.56 and 5.67, respectively. Data from *Selected Educational Statistics* of the Ministry of Human Resource Development, which is also given by Mary John in her analysis, show that in 2006–7 the GER for men in the age group 18–23 was 11.1 (made up of 7.8 million degree and diploma holders in a population of 70 million), while for women the comparable figure was 7.9 (4.95 million women in a population of 62 million) (John 2008: 57).
7. Engineers and nurses are an interesting comparison, especially on points of educational decision-making and status as they epitomise the masculine and feminine professions, respectively.
8. Mariamma's comment highlights the absence of parents from the educational decision-making scenario of their children. It shows that access to information on nursing education was available even to someone whose family could not provide it for her.
9. The professionalism and service conditions of J.J. hospital and Shanti Mukand (in Delhi) where she was working at the time of the interview cannot be compared. That struck me as odd and I later found that she had left her nursing job a few years after her marriage to a pastor. She started working again to support herself and her children after some marital discord. At the time of the interview, her husband was in Kerala while she, with her two children, decided to stay on in Delhi.
10. Also, the comparison between a secretarial job and nursing made by Annamma in the previous chapter becomes relevant. As a choice, however, this does not come up unlike school teaching.
11. *Times of India*, 'When Nurses are Muslims…', 19 December 2008, p. 9 (http://articles.timesofindia.indiatimes.com/2006-12-17/india/27813741_1_nursing-schools-muslims-girls-profession.
12. In fact, Delhi hospital administrators distinguish Malayali nurses from the local ones by describing the former as submissive and praise them as natural carers because of this aspect, which some others describe as mediocre and lacking in initiative. While it is true that professionals who work in life-saving situations have to be team players, assuming that a woman would be naturally caring and would be willing to take orders is cultural to a great extent.

Many institutions state the other qualities too, for example, the need to communicate well and handle non-cooperative patients.

13. My pilot study on women at the graduate level, engineering educational institutions in Kerala and Rajasthan done in 2010–11 shows that specialisations in engineering are gendered and categorised as suitable and unsuitable for women. For pilot study, see unpublished report titled 'Women in Indian Engineering', A Report from the Graduate Level Engineering Education Field in Kerala and Rajasthan at the CWDS and Centre des Sciences Humaines, New Delhi. It can also be accessed at the CWDS library. Also see 'What It Takes To Be A Woman Engineer by Sreelekha Nair', WFS REF NO: INDk721f.

14. http://articles.timesofindia.indiatimes.com/2006-12-17/india/27813741_1_nursing-school-muslim-girls-profession.

15. Ibid.

16. In fact, even while the participation of women outside the home is encouraged, their primary identity as wives and mothers and thus secondary to men in the public space was reinforced. Anna Lindberg's study (2001) of the cashew industry, for example, discusses how the idea of family wages relegated women's right to full wages as unimportant by trade unions, even while fighting for women workers' rights to maternity benefits.

17. The sentence is highlighted to draw attention of the readers to the manner in which care is described by individual nurses.

18. Sexual harassment case against Mr T.V. Rama Rao, Andhra Pradesh MLA that came out in the press on 14 June 2009 is a notorious example. Five girls from Kerala who were studying in the nursing school run by him in the West Godavari district alleged sexual harassment and threats by the MLA.

19. Hilda Lazarus, an Indian doctor at Christian Medical College (CMC), Vellore, and the first Indian woman Chief Medical Officer of the Women's Medical Service in 1947, known to have made significant contributions to medicine and nursing in India, remarked in a pamphlet for the All India Women's Conference about nurses that: 'Their task was arduous and irksome ... The strain was great, and when temptation came in the guise of a kind invitation from a generous-hearted man, it was accepted.... Repeated invitations came, she could not resist the temptation and she fell—a ruined woman, a greater outcast in Society, the finger pointed at her. Was the profession such! How could any self-respecting parents countenance their daughters going in for nursing or midwifery!'

20. Quoted from Nair and Healey (2006: 14).

4

Migration

Delhi as a Transit Residence

Migration is an inevitable step once one selects nursing as a profession. Migrating to Delhi is part of a 'big' and elongated plan for the future that stretches beyond. As Table 4.1 suggests, 114 of the sample in the study planned further migration, while all of them considered moving to pursue better opportunities as normal. While 36 of them considered themselves as without any solid plans of migration, they would not miss any future opportunity without serious consideration. Of them three had gone abroad (to countries in the Persian Gulf) for work and returned. Their migration narrative places India as offering them a better life situation despite its poor working conditions than the countries where they worked. What is striking is that even when they do not have a plan to migrate, their lives in Delhi are informed by the migration trajectory.

The recent literature on women's migration for work emphasises the importance of looking at how women's decisions are formed as much by the opportunities at home as by those at the new place (Agrawal 2006: 21–45; Barber 2000: 402; Harzig 2001: 15–28[1]). Nurses take initiatives to find out through networks and other sources as much as possible by comparing different destinations before making a decision. Though this is relevant to men as well, physical security is a special and compulsory concern for women migrants, often taking first priority in their enquiries[2] about their destination. Nurses migrating from Kerala to different Indian cities usually have no job in hand but find one in a few weeks' time. This is because of easy availability of nursing jobs due to the shortage of nurses in private hospitals. Their networks help them find jobs, which, in most cases, are not advertised. In my study there were only four cases from Kerala out of the total of 150 who had applied for

TABLE 4.1

Respondents and their Migration Plans

	Age	With migration plan	No current migration plan	Total
	22–25	54	2	56
	26–30	57	12	69
	31–35	3	10	13
	36–40	–	7	7
	41–45	–	3	3
	46–50	–	1	1
	51–55	–	1	1
Total	22–55	114	36	150

Note: One each from among the age group of 26–30, 36–40 and 46–50 had her migration spelt out. All of them had worked as staff nurses in hospitals in the Gulf.

Source: Data collected from respondents through questionnaire and interview.

jobs in Delhi in response to newspaper advertisements; they were directly employed in government hospitals. A few others who came to Delhi looking for work in other fields were also subsequently trained as nurses.[3] Many nurses told me that it is possible to find employment in Delhi hospitals within two weeks of applying. This may be the reason why 7,500[4] Malayali nurses are working in Delhi hospitals. However, this possibility of finding a job quickly applies only to private hospitals, since government hospitals follow formal recruitment procedures like inviting applications through newspaper advertisements and interviews.

Barrie Morrison's study (1997) of three villages in Kerala in the 1990s casts some insights into migration as a strategy adopted by (male) members of rural communities in Kerala as the aftermath of investing in education as part of diversifying their sources of income. Though this study is conspicuous by the absence of any reference to a trained nurse in any of the three villages,[5] his analyses apply to the processes of movement-seeking work by the latter category as well. He says that the following are compulsory for successful migration: '...skills that were saleable in the distant job market; money to pay for the trip and the job search (estimated at ₹50,000 for a Gulf migrant); connections into the target community; the help and reassurance from the returned migrants or "role models"' (p. 78).

In almost every case of nurses applying for jobs after reaching Delhi, their decisions were guided by the factors put forth by Morrison above. In fact, travelling to Delhi, a strange city where they would be completely dependent on their networks, is said to have been mostly due to financial considerations. As mentioned earlier in the chapter on nursing education, nurses seek information on salary and technical advancement, possibility of attending coaching classes for CGFNS and IELTS that facilitate further migration before relying on their networks to reach Delhi. They do acquire this information through seniors, colleagues and friends during their stay in the nursing school.

Delhi formed the centre of a migration plan to popular destinations like the US, UK and the Gulf countries. The Gulf countries, though not the first priority destination, are seen as a stepping stone towards the ultimate objective of reaching the West. The hierarchy of destinations is decided after evaluation of standards of living, life chances, availability of citizenship and possibilities of buying property. Arrangements for direct movement to western countries by some of the affluent nurses are pointed out as 'money-power' by some respondents. For those who come to Delhi, the experiences of working in a hospital, the training in various sections within the hospital and the language skills are important. They also heed the advice and wisdom shared by friends or relatives in whose residence they initially stay. These friends, neighbours and relatives form the most vital link between Delhi and their homes in Kerala and thus form a predominantly female network. The role of networks has also been emphasised in much of the general literature on migration.[6] Once they are in Delhi, they also rely on formal mechanisms and institutions to migrate, like the recruitment agencies, and yet vetting these agencies through their networks saves them trouble in some cases.

Delhi comes out as a place of immense importance in shaping their future plans even if they had pre-decided their migration abroad. Delhi is also 'not a bad place to stay on if migration plans fail' according to Sheila, who came to Delhi to study analytical chemistry, but subsequently left the course to become a nurse. She had gone to the Gulf but returned to stay on in Delhi and was in the process of deciding and finalising her migration plans back to Kerala 'where she had started it all'. Some nurses in my study stayed on, not because they had abandoned their migration plans forever but because of concerns over their children's education, satisfaction over work conditions, the inability to convince their families about moving again, and uncertainty over the future. Public sector employment[7] in itself is no guarantee for satisfaction and in such cases, reportedly, the only difference is that they think harder before going abroad, as in the case of Sindhu discussed earlier. I illustrate the cases of three nurses ahead to show how Delhi figures in their lives. These examples inform us of the real life situations and challenges faced by these women in a city like Delhi.

Diana

The first case is that of Diana who earns ₹140,000 annually on a salary scale of ₹5,500–5,800 as a staff nurse in Sir Ganga Ram Hospital in Karol Bagh. This is after eight years of work experience. Her first move out of Kerala was for her nursing studies. She went to Ongole, Andhra Pradesh, for her GNM course and came to Delhi through a 'family connection'—with her aunt (mother's sister). Her aunt works in a public sector company and has settled in Delhi with her family (her husband works in the same company and she has two children). Diana worked in Mata Channan Devi, a private charitable hospital in west Delhi for four years before joining Sir Ganga Ram Hospital where she has been working since 2000.

She would have loved to get a 'good' nursing job in Kerala (meaning with a good salary and working conditions). Yet it was on the cards that she had to go elsewhere to work. Migration was, therefore, on her mind when she started enquiring about nursing studies, and this is not anything extraordinary, according to her. When she got the job with Sir Ganga Ram Hospital, she was satisfied and thought that her coming to Delhi was a success. This is a story that was repeated many times over during my interview, that is, nurses' satisfaction with an individual hospital which makes them view their migration to Delhi as a success.

Diana described her life in Delhi at length, including how her parents and relatives in Delhi found her a suitable marriage alliance in the city. She described her decisions to work, marry and settle down in Delhi as well-thought-out decisions, on the basis of direct knowledge about the arduous trajectories older cousins of her generation had gone through. A male cousin had done an MA in Kerala and then married a girl who was a nurse in Switzerland. They subsequently shifted to Austria when they learnt about the better salary options there from the wife of another cousin. However, the husband could not find a good job. Meanwhile, he did a nursing course in Austria and they returned to Switzerland where he went on to start a business in medical equipment. They offered to help her join them but she was not ready to face the uncertainty of a foreign land.

Diana graduated in economics, not knowing what to study next in order to get a job. She ended up studying nursing in Andhra Pradesh (non-science students cannot study nursing in Kerala). She first tried to find different nursing schools in the neighbouring Indian states, especially Andhra Pradesh, Karnataka and Tamil Nadu—and in that order of importance. Andhra Pradesh was the first preference for Diana as it has a large number of nursing schools with numerous Malayali students. She and her family chose one that asked for the lowest donation (₹10,000), fees and hostel charges. The donation was lower than in other reputed schools in Andhra Pradesh. Considering that nursing is free and nursing students get a stipend to cover their expenses during their studies, her family thought that ₹10,000 to be a large sum; her family could not have afforded more than that. Though hostel and other facilities during the studies were well organised, it soon became clear to her that Andhra Pradesh was not the place for a job, as the wages and standards of hospital service are very low. There are many nursing students attached to nursing schools, leading to an over supply of nurses. Technological advancements in Delhi are also plus points compared to hospitals in Kerala or small towns elsewhere in India. In her mind, probably only Mumbai has better hospitals.

Since Diana's aunt was willing to bring her to Delhi, she came without hesitation. Since physical safety was the primary concern for the family, she felt lucky to have an aunt in Delhi who was ready to accommodate her. She first stayed with her aunt for five to six months and then joined a friend in a rented place. Then she stayed in the Mata Channan Devi hostel for a year (in 1999) when her roommate, who was also a nurse, left to work in a hospital in Kuwait. When she joined Sir Ganga Ram

Hospital, she joined other friends in their accommodation near Karol Bagh till she got married.

Diana's main problem in Delhi was language. She found herself unable to converse either in English with the doctors or in Hindi with the patients and others. She had managed to get through her training by speaking a mix of Malayalam and English; by the time I met her she managed to speak some English though not very fluently. Feeling inadequate because she was unable to converse with the majority of the patients and hospital staff due to her lack of fluency in Hindi, she discussed the issue with nursing friends and decided to speak only in Hindi with them. Her Malayali senior colleagues always spoke to her in Hindi and helped her by insisting that she should speak in Hindi even when she made mistakes. They made her stay comfortable in the initial days in many ways. She did not find it difficult to rent accommodation when she wanted to move out of her aunt's place because of help from her colleagues. She wanted to stay only with nurses from her hospital and there were many who would have kept her as their roommate.

Diana describes the local Hindi-speaking population as generally friendly, but also very calculating. While staying in Janakpuri, she was singled out in a hostile situation in a shop in Tilak Nagar market—'*yeh pardeshi hei*' (this is an outsider) said an old woman in a heavy Punjabi accent. Diana was unable to explain her side of the story, and found the vulnerability of single women in such situations agonising. She felt helpless because she could not respond properly in Hindi. The incident made her determined to learn Hindi and not tolerate such 'nonsense' in future (she laughs). Here one can see her enhanced confidence and an implicit sense of entitlement over Delhi as a shared city for everyone in India, and not a north Indian city. Yet, she has had to learn to live with the fact that she is a migrant and does not truly belong.

> I too have (an) equal right to this place like anyone else (but) I do not think much on those lines...especially to keep my peace of mind. It is not the thing to dwell on. I have my family here now and a child to look after. So long as no one is bothered about me living here, I am not going to make it a big issue... I do reply to people when they say something that I do not like. While I am part of the Malayali population in Delhi I realise I am not a part of the

whole city…But you know one is busy just trying to do one's job…
Where is the time (to bother about such things)? … In that sense
everyone is so busy; no one is part of anyone's life here…

Experiencing isolation, she tries to identify with the Malayalis
in the city. There is also the loneliness she feels in the anonymity of a busy life. She tries to keep in touch with other Malayalis
by participating in festivals like Onam (the harvest festival of
Kerala) and through regular visits to the church on Sundays.
She goes regularly for morning mass on Sundays except when
she has night shifts. While life in Delhi is busy, she prefers it
to the one in Kerala where, she says, interference is the norm.
People in Kerala have too much time to gossip about others'
lives and so it is better to be cut off and limit oneself to one's
own life in Delhi.

Diana believes that the rich and poor people in Delhi, and
also elsewhere, have different approaches towards nurses. The
attitude of the rich patients is detestable. They do not respect
the advice given to them and expect nurses to treat them differently from other common patients. That, along with the night
shifts, is her main problem with a nursing job. The situation is
made more complicated because the locals think that nurses
from Kerala migrate due to poverty. My queries about possible
collective action are met with disinterest. In case of a problem
she will just approach the Staff Welfare Board that is part of
the grievance redressal mechanism for the staff in Sir Ganga
Ram Hospital, which does not allow an employees' union. She
believes that nurses alone cannot change their status or salary.
Nurses are not respected much within the hospital either, but
then Kerala is no different. At the end of our discussion she
confides that she will leave the hospital should a 'really big'
problem arise rather than fighting the authorities. There is no
point worsening relations with one's employers by arguing over
small matters. She explains that it is not bad at present because
jobs are readily available in Delhi, and, with so many years of
experience, one can always get a better one.

Her husband (with a degree in hotel management) works as an
assistant manager in a private hotel. No one else in her immediate family has taken up nursing. Her sisters work as accountants
in private companies in Kerala. She has a one-and-a-half year
old son. It was interesting that she first discussed her personal life

with me, after all the references to the pastime of gossip. Though she had first said she had had an arranged marriage, she later changed her story thus indicating greater trust in me by revealing her perceptions of what is acceptable and ideal. She admitted that she had not told anyone that she had known her husband before their marriage out of fear that they would cast aspersions on her character. She and her husband met in a church in Delhi and they decided to get married. Once that decision was made, he met her parents. The two families belonged to the same religious denomination and had the same socio-economic status. There was no opposition to the marriage from either family. She has a maid from Bihar to help her at home and to look after her son. Nuclear family or not, there is a change in the attitude towards young wives in Delhi and other metros, she feels. Her husband considers her opinion before deciding on important matters, which she considers as having an equal status in the relationship. Her night shifts are respected by her family and are seen as more difficult than the day shifts.

There has been a cooling in her relationship with her relatives. Once she decided to settle in Delhi she felt less interested in maintaining relations that are not primary in nature. Before marriage, she sent all her earnings to her parents with no idea of what they did with the money. After her marriage she no longer sends money; instead, she gives plenty of clothes and electronic goods as gifts when visiting her parents once a year. However, she does not take anything for her relatives because they are not satisfied with the gifts she brings and she realises that she cannot satiate their requirements.

Bindu

Unlike Diana, Bindu had certain predetermined and specific plans on nursing. Bindu migrated to Jhansi, Uttar Pradesh, for her GNM course. She possessed all the academic qualifications to get admission in a nursing school in Kerala but could not pass the entrance examination. When she got it in a private Christian nursing school, she could not afford the ₹ 50,000 donation demanded for admission. So she applied to the same nursing school in Jhansi where her sister was studying; her sister had heard about it from a nun in the local school and one of her Christian neighbours. When Bindu got the call, she went to

Uttar Pradesh with her sister. One of her older sisters works as a staff nurse in Lucknow, and she has older female cousins working as nurses in Amethi in Uttar Pradesh and Haryana, thus providing her with a fairly good idea of what to expect in north India as far as nursing was concerned.

When Bindu finished her GNM course she stayed with her cousin in Amethi before shifting to Delhi. Delhi, she felt, gave more exposure and is modern. This job in Sir Ganga Ram Hospital came through a newspaper advertisement.

When I met Bindu she had already worked out her life in Delhi, month by month for the coming year, so as to facilitate her plan to migrate to the UK or US. There are training centres for the English language[8] in Delhi and hospitals there are equipped with the latest technology in medical care. 'It adds to your CV if you work in a better hospital', she affirmed. Unlike Diana, her plan to go abroad kept her focussed on her goals and her interaction with local people was minimum. She liked to spend her time studying and planning about her and her family's future.

Her sisters did not really want to be nurses and it was the persuasion of a Christian neighbour that made one of them join. This particular neighbour had three daughters in nursing who were earning well. But in her sisters' minds, and for her parents, nursing was taken up in conditions of extreme adversity and poverty. Now, while her Hindu neighbours opt for nursing, the stigma has not gone away, even after many among the 'upper castes' have taken it up as a profession. The local population looks down on nurses in particular because of their different lifestyle. By this she means the migration, kind of married life, etc., very different from the 'norm' in Kerala. The norm in Kerala, according to Bindu, is that a woman is primarily responsible for her family. And if she is a working woman, ideally she should be home by 5 pm. According to Bindu these reasons make it tough for nurses to get married in Kerala.

Her only regular contacts beyond work are with the Malayali nurses with whom she stays, and with her family. She does not go to the temple or to any festivals organised by different Malayali groups. But Bindu complains of loneliness even when she is with nurses in a homely atmosphere. She finds Sir Ganga Ram Hospital better than the other hospitals where she initially worked, in Amethi and in Jhansi, in that the atmosphere is more cosmopolitan and the staff more technically advanced and skilful. But the patients are from a higher income bracket and are more suspicious of nurses' competence and refuse to obey nurses' orders. They are educated and more informed and demanding of nurses than of doctors, while the rural setting in Uttar Pradesh was more laid back, the facilities were minimal and patients simpler.

As pointed out in the chapter on educational choices, her decision to take up nursing was completely due to the sense of duty she felt towards her family. She was clear about her financial responsibility as far as her parents and brother are concerned. She saves money from her salary to help her father who is ill and needs medical interventions at regular intervals. Her sisters are married and her brother, who is a professional visual artist, is not in a position to earn much. Her father is a heart patient and their house was built with a bank loan. Moreover, she has to save for her own marriage expenses, which, according to her, would be substantial. But marriage is not part of her immediate plans. Her priority is to migrate to the West, since that is the only way to overcome the family's financial problems. Moreover, in order to (re)gain her understanding of herself as successful and as someone who works hard, she looks at migration to a western country as a solution. Yet she worries about going far away from her home because her father is sick and she would like to be closer.

> ...I was always good in studies and nursing was not the thing I would have opted for if I were rich... (It would have been something) that brings in a sense of achievement that (I) otherwise miss in nursing. I am not particularly unhappy about being a nurse but that is not enough. I want to do as much as I can...I would have been a good doctor if I could; but I am a nurse. I want to do everything that will make my family's position better. Only thing is that I cannot do all these if I am in Kerala... I miss my family. I want to be near my father who is a heart patient. I am worried about my brother's progress in his career. I don't mind drawing as and when I have time. (But) I think that it is better to pursue it as a hobby because I have to have a stable income from a salaried job...

Bindu is proud that she got a first division throughout her studies, a distinction (more than 80 per cent marks) in grade 10, and wants to look at other options while earning her salary. She was in fact the only one who asked me about the details of my PhD in Sociology and wanted to know about courses offered in the Centre for Social Medicine and Community Health in Jawaharlal Nehru University, New Delhi. I collected all the information for her as she said she wanted to do an MPhil in community health. However, when I met her six months later she said she had dropped the idea of doing her MPhil because she could not afford to attend classes regularly.

Bindu now shares her flat with four Malayali nurses. Three of them are preparing for an English language test that will make them eligible to apply for work in the West, whereas the fourth is going to appear for an interview for a job in a government hospital in Saudi Arabia. Overall, her plans to be a nurse and to migrate are connected to her family's well being. Her affection towards her brother came out in every sentence. Considering that he is older than her, she seems determined to act as the one responsible for the family so that he can pursue his dream as an artist while she, who also draws well, let go of hers.

Beena Jacob

Beena studied in Bengaluru when it was called Bangalore. Her stated reason to come to Delhi to work as a staff nurse was to improve her language, mainly English but Hindi as well. She paid ₹40,000 as a donation to get admission to Dr Shyamala Reddy School of Nursing in Bangalore. She sends money home every month after covering her expenses and preparations for her later migration and said that she is not saving for dowry or marriage expenses which are her parents' responsibility.

Beena chose nursing because she felt it offered her job opportunities and a chance to serve sick people. Friends helped her come to Delhi since she was not happy with the working conditions and salary in Bangalore. And her former classmates and friends in Delhi offered solutions. Kerala was not an option as the salary offered in private hospitals was too low.

> ...Moreover once you are outside Kerala, you do not feel like returning there [smiles]. Life opportunities expand when you are

in a big city but in Kerala no one knows what happens beyond their houses and neighbourhood. If I want to join a course, I have to travel more than 30 kilometres to reach the nearest town and it is very tiring too; [somehow the] motivation to do anything like that is very low when I am in Kerala... And if it rains, my mother would say 'do not go today'. Here I meet my friends and we make plans, share everything and study together. My housemates are very helpful. We all have a dream to go to the US or the UK...And here everyone—doctors, other nurses and the general public —understands our ambition to be something...In Kerala people make fun of me if I say that I want to go to the US...They (seem to) think that I cannot go there...

Her father's sister was the first to join nursing and some of her cousins have also joined nursing. On arriving in Delhi, she first stayed with her friends' sisters and then with nurse friends who were working in the same hospital. She prefers the lifestyle, climate and cleanliness of Bangalore, but Delhi clearly offers more opportunities.

It is interesting that though they stay together and work at the same place, the four nurses' opinions on issues are different though not poles apart. Beena finds that there is a clear discrimination towards nurses within hospitals and outside. Character assassination and contempt towards each other based on family background is common in work situations and even in their personal lives. Delhi offers better treatment than Kerala. But she also feels that people change their views after they have interacted closely and are also more educated. That is why she believes that status issues are not a major issue.

Earlier Beena used to be homesick but has adjusted to a very different way of life. Her main contact with Malayalis is through the church which she visits regularly. She does not mingle with locals outside the hospital and cannot say anything about them but yes, as nurses, there is a problem when it comes to local people. She was not ready to specify the nature of the problem to me. For her, it was not important to know what the local population is like because she was 'not going to stay here'. Beena's opinion was that Delhi hospitals are much better workplaces than those of Kerala and hence she did not see the point in complaining.

From these examples from the lives of my respondents it is clear that factors like language and a place to carry out their plans for the future are prominent factors in the process of migration. These take the form of recurring themes. Questions related to family, decisions over nursing as a profession, job opportunities, future plans, and friends and/or family members who are nurses are all interconnected and smoothly flow into each other. Yet it is clear that these happen in a phased manner and that considerable planning has gone into the process of reaching Delhi. Feelings of being treated unfairly appear in the interviews with all nurses though their responses to such experiences differ based on their individual experiences and perceptions of the choices available.

Social Networks: 'There are Malayali Nurses in all the Hospitals in Delhi'[9]

Leela Gulati (1993) has explored how networks operate in the case of male migrants from Kerala to the west Asian 'Gulf' countries. She finds that there are various instrumentalities associated with such networks, which include relatives, friends and neighbours. Mobilising funds and obtaining work permits are the major tasks achieved through networks, which bypass expensive recruiting agents. She has discussed the expectations for reciprocity that arise out of the help that is provided to the migrants. Silvey and Elmhirst (2003: 2), in the context of rural urban Indonesia, argue that social networks help us understand the complexities of the processes of migration beyond the state and the market, and certainly beyond the limited assumptions of neo-classical migration theory. According to them, social networks draw on an individual's social capital and cushion a person from collapse at times of economic crisis. Such an approach, however, is limited in explaining the non-economic advantages of networks and in a certain sense polarises the discourse around the gendered access to resources. Silvey and Elmhirst conclude that gender-specific networks disadvantage women by excluding them from the powerful networks that men form. However, this line of argument does not consider that social capital itself is gendered in its origin and distribution and that it could not be differently managed through networks, since ideologies of allocation of social capital remain the same.[10] Yet there are some advantages that women-specific networks offer. Percot's study (2005) discusses the context of Keralite migration to West Asian countries of the Persian Gulf where there is an unstated expectation of 'return' favours by male migrants, which is often translated into tangible benefits in monetary terms and gifts. Sometimes this expectation takes the form of assisting in the migration of a family member at a later moment. There are also explicit forms of competition among male migrants, especially among unskilled labourers. This, Percot states, contrasts with the helpful all-female networks of migrant Malayali nurses, leading to strong suggestions of the gendered nature of networking. Other narrations of women seeking work elsewhere also illustrate the presence of networks of female migrants based on nationality and language and the interlocking of concerns of work with marriage and so on.

My study questions gender-blind models of networking. Nurses' networks are constituted by inter- and intra-household power dynamics over family resources, which affect the very choice of this profession. Here, the exclusivity of women's networks provides them with the space to make their own decisions, and this space seems to be one of the compensations they expect while conforming to gender norms otherwise. It is also interesting that these networks often do the 'chaperoning' required in a patriarchal society like that of Kerala.

Though no one-to-one favours were expressed among my respondents, there were complaints about the 'thanklessness' of certain relatives, friends and neighbours who had been helped during their initial months of settling down in Delhi. There is, however, nothing typically 'feminine' about this as men are also heard to complain of lack of contact from those whom they have helped. These are spaces of negotiation of hierarchies, of power and control, and, to some extent, reveal intergenerational variations in the understanding of social relations, assistance and gratitude. For example, Susanna Koshi (44 years old) says that sometimes Malayali nurses avoid keeping in touch with those who helped them relocate to Delhi.

> I have brought my relatives... my husband's relatives... many of them to Delhi. [I] Went around Delhi looking for jobs according to their qualification...which you know, as those who stay in Delhi know, is not easy; it is a big place not like your typical

Kerala town. They talk of Delhi as if it is the centre of a town but it is a big place; it is a state and the weather can be very harsh. Finally, when they get jobs they don't even smile back at us... boys are better... they at least visit us once a while and ask how I am doing; how uncle is doing, etc... for Onam, Christmas. I have this [nurse] niece of my husband... you know I got her the job on contract but in a government hospital... it was not easy... I really talked to a lot of people before she got that job. Now she does not even call ...even for Christmas or New Year...I am not complaining but I know that these young nurses have a different outlook; they look out for chances to go abroad...nothing about the family...Forget about me!

The discourse on reciprocity and consequent expectations makes it seem as if there is no way for those who have received favours to return them or express their gratitude, since any attempt to do so is perceived as inadequate, while 'no attempt' to do so is seen as thanklessness. It thus becomes a Catch-22 situation for new migrants. Nevertheless, minimal expectations include keeping in touch through phone calls at regular intervals and occasional visits.

As shown in the earlier discussion on nursing school experiences, nurses' social networks develop around a nucleus of nursing schools, job opportunities, migration possibilities and competitive examinations like IELTS and CGFNS. Relying on this social network is completely normal. As a matter of fact, it would be 'abnormal' if anyone was to 'show independence' and bypass such networks or refuse to acknowledge them. Interestingly, one way to show disapproval of a nurse is to say, 'She does not even talk to other Malayalis'. Contrary to the positive experiences of networking, there is much grumbling in government hospitals over Malayali nurses who are not friendly and who do not recognise other Malayalis.

As Sally told me in another context about a Malayali nurse who passed us when we were halfway through the interview:

...normally we are all very helpful, generous and good to each other... If someone tries to show that she does not need any help, fine, go ahead but it is not necessary to flex muscles to show us that...There is so much more you can do if you are 'naturally' friendly[11]...

By the end of their term as students, each nurse seems to be well-entrenched in some 'group' or the other composed of class-mates who discuss fashion, cinema and songs, as well as friends and cousins (who are invariably men and any mention of them produces blushes, smirks and meaningful glances from others in the group). Fashion, cinema and songs are three spheres that clearly exemplify their lives at the interface between Kerala and Delhi. They not only illustrate their evolving tastes and preferences, but also demonstrate the sense of balance they are supposed to maintain between the two cultures in which they live. At one end are the laudable myths around Kerala film stars like Mammootty, Mohanlal and Dileep and on the other the heroics of Bollywood stars like Shahrukh Khan or the beauty of Aishwarya Rai. Tamil movies are also discussed, sometimes in detail. Movie dialogues often form a part of arguments on issues and constitute entertainment for groups during leisure time. In the context of masculine styles and movie heroes in Kerala, Osella and Osella (2006: 199) say that '...young men repeat *dialogue* and copy hairstyles, follow *cinema* fashions and modify their walks, they maintain a sense that this is all play, a matter of aesthetics and surfaces'. This is what is on display with the women who traverse the path of multicultural, linguistic exposure to film watching and real life.

Through their contacts, as seen, these groups learn about job possibilities, advancements in the profession and migration opportunities in hospitals and cities. They share the cost of long-distance phone calls and expenses like food on train journeys. Reserving train tickets on the Kerala Express from Kerala to Delhi is the first step and the number of friends leaving together is finalised. Travelling in a group is preferred but even two friends leaving together is common. This avoids the anxiety of parents who feel the need to accompany single girls to Delhi. For example, Shijy George said her father accompanied her sister and her to make sure that they faced no problem during their journey to Delhi and while settling down. She said she was confident of making it alone and, in any case, her sister was travelling with her. But she thinks that her father was almost tyrannical in his control of his daughters, which she resented.

> ...He came with us to Moolchand Hospital [she was in Jaipur Golden when I was interviewing her]...My sister joined Batra

Hospital. My father left us only after we went inside the hostels. That created a funny scene as well because that day he made [a] ruckus at the reception of the hospital's hostel by insisting that he had to see the hostel room before he left and hostel rules did not allow that. No male visitors are allowed inside...

But this seems to have been an extreme case of concern by Shijy's own admission. Parents and often the entire family reach the railway station to see the girl off. They bring packed bags for the three-day train journey with clothes and food. Bottled pickles, chips (banana, tapioca and jackfruit)—for the girls and for friends, relatives and neighbours whom they are going to meet in Delhi—fill the bags. Friends and relatives then reach New Delhi railway station to receive them and to take them home. Many in my study venture out to apply for a job the very next day. Much depends on the convenience of the friend/relative who has to take them around. Sonia, Reeja and Rani, for example, went with Sonia's aunt who was working as a senior nurse in a large public hospital. They went to a private hospital and applied for the post of staff nurse by submitting plain paper applications, and waited till the aunt finished her duty at 2.30 pm. Then they went to five different hospitals and nursing homes. All of them were appointed within two weeks and were happy to be able to shift to the hostels of the respective hospitals.

Thus, migration is as normal and intrinsic an aspect of life for a nurse as going to school is. The associated activities of migration provide the appearance of a straightforward activity, while concealing several knotty procedures. The physical process of migration can be usefully broken up into several stages and moves, starting with the decision to take up nursing which involves planning all decisions about the future.

As we have seen, ethnic, gender and professional identities of Malayali nurses play the most important part in the creation of these informal networks consisting of female classmates, friends, relatives and neighbours. Most of these women leave home with an inherent faith in the helpfulness of these networks at various stages of their operation. That is why the statement by one of the respondents that 'there are a large number of Malayalis in Delhi and that there is no hospital in the world where there is no Malayali nurse' becomes solid ground for these women to venture out to Delhi in the first place. This confidence comes from stories they have heard about decades-old migration to various parts of the country and even abroad. The aura of success surrounding such narratives is part of the topic of migration in Kerala.

Migrants never fail! Every migrant goes to places where milk and honey flows. This orientation places immense pressure on the migrants to perform under adverse situations. The cases of a few Delhi nurses who went through extreme adversity in this study illustrate that even relatively well-educated nurse migrants, in comparison to domestic workers and unskilled labour, are by no means exempt from negative outcomes. Two women found ways of coping by converting to another religion that offered sympathy and suggested solutions to their problems, which included sheer poverty and marital breakdowns. In all these cases they saw no hope in returning to Kerala either.

Failed cases of migration are not taken lightly. There are numerous examples of failed male migrations to Delhi and to the Gulf countries by men who could not cope with the pressures of a new place. Many who return, unsuccessful, are mocked by neighbours and relatives.[12] The harsh climate, strange customs, language and anonymity of the large city are significant factors that can provoke migrants to rethink their decision. It is specifically at those moments of self-doubt that the image of the faceless yet sympathetic Malayali population comes to everyone's mind.

Jalaja, 32 years old at the time of the interview, who attended but could not complete her GNM course in Kerala, migrated to Delhi with her married sister who was working in a factory in the Mayapuri industrial area. She too soon started working in a factory in Naraina. The economic situation was bad and Jalaja's language skills were not good either. She started going to the Pentecostal church on the advice of a friend when she fell ill. She had a continuous stomach ache and fever for several months. Collective prayers were organised for her health and she soon found herself back in a stable health situation. She started going regularly to the church and converted to the Pentecostal denomination. Her family was against the decision but she felt that 'it was a calling'.[13] Later, she married her friend's brother, a motor vehicle mechanic with a very unstable job, who worked in a shop near the CRPF camp in Vikaspuri. At the time of the interview, he had lost his job with a private company on a monthly salary as he had refused a transfer to a village in Uttar Pradesh.

Saradamoni (1995: 157) has described the case of seasonal Malayali women migrants to the Gujarat fishing sector, showing how these 'women do not always leave with a job arranged. They go along with friends or relatives or travel alone and then seek work upon arrival'. While nurses share similar experiences about leaving home without a fixed job, they have very concrete hopes of support in terms of the numerous Malayali nurses who would help them get a job on arrival. They are very certain about the popularity of Malayali nurses and, hence, of their job chances.

Shylaja's words represent the general idea:

> ...I knew that I would get a job in any of the hospitals in Delhi. Moreover my friends reassured me that they would find me a job where they worked and that it was better than not having a job and staying home in Kerala. After all I did my GNM for a job...

Reena adds:

> Is there any hospital in Delhi which does not have a Malayali nurse?... Impossible...The majority of [Malayali] women migrants are nurses and ...Even in this area [Rohini Sector 3] where I stay, the highest number of women [Malayalis] are nurses.

While this confidence does help these women make the move to relocate to Delhi, nurses in government hospitals in Delhi say that this trend is beginning to reverse. This is discussed in further detail later. Nonetheless, the 'omnipresent', soft, compassionate and docile Malayali nurse is a popular figure not just in the minds of the general public but also among the nurses themselves. Their reported docility is seen as feminine and an appropriate quality for nurses.

Stay in hostels and homes: 'The new girl needs a place to live'

Nurses from Kerala cluster around certain localities and form what can informally be called 'neighbourhoods'. These clusters are near hospitals and are sometimes characterised by the presence of large numbers of migrant Malayalis, many of whom are non-nurses. But what characterises nurses' clusters in particular is that they are often inhabited by single women who work in the same hospital. These areas become identified as 'safe and friendly' for nurses and are then recommended to new migrants. Local people and shopkeepers become sociable and even start learning a few words in Malayalam, interacting with them in a jovial manner. These interactions are the windows to the local society where reciprocal exchanges on the culture and habits of the southern and northern parts of the country are learnt in bits and pieces through *idli* and *dosa* making, and the knitting of woollen sweaters, giving an opportunity to bust or buttress the stereotypes of 'Madrasi' and 'Punjabi'. Malayali grocery shops too emerge over a period of time. One nurse brought her brother to one such cluster in which she was living and he started a small tea shop there, much as it exists in Kerala. As these rooms and clusters are safe for nurses, especially those assumed to be single, Christian women from Kerala, the rents in these clusters are hiked periodically. However, nurses also say that there is a decline in the number of such neighbourhoods because more and more hospitals and nursing homes have started offering hostel accommodation, whose facilities have improved.

A visit to the hostels, however, disillusioned me. Rooms are anything but spacious. Except for Ganga Ram, Apollo and government hospitals, the rest provide hostel facilities that are clearly sub-standard. Some nurses' hostels are in separate blocs within the hospital compound and some are above the wards themselves. Most of the private hospitals rent flats in residential areas, allotting a room each to three to five nurses with a common kitchen and toilet-bathroom. In some hostels, big halls are partitioned as rooms using curtains, but with no further privacy. Cooking gas cylinders and accommodation are free, but house rent is deducted from the salary. Free movement is only allowed from 7 am to 7 or 8 pm.[14] Nurses have to sign a register kept at the entrance and provide details of their personal trips including shopping. One of the senior nurses is put in charge of the hostel and is called the matron or warden, and is supposed to monitor the movements of the women residents. Male visitors are strictly not allowed. Cooking is managed collectively. Quarrels regarding favourite vegetables, fish, meat and who should cook what, how many times a week and so on are frequent but the more assertive women get away with what they want.

Hospitals are invariably at an advantage here for two reasons. First, hostel arrangements are cost-effective. Second, they are able to control the movements of the nurses even outside the hospitals by providing the hospital ambulance for their transport whenever necessary for duty. Travel allowance ceases to be the concern of the hospital management whether the hostels are within the compound or not when ambulances are provided for transport. It also helps the hospitals employ nurses for extra hours even after work in case of emergencies or if someone on duty goes on leave.

For example, a medium-sized hospital in east Delhi, sent the ambulance driver to pick up the night shift nurses from the hostel. On arriving, the driver blew his horn to indicate to the nurses they had to come downstairs soon. Due to some confusion, the women were not ready and they thought that the driver had come early. When the ever-enthusiastic Rani went down to investigate, it turned out that the ambulance was indeed early. Later, when speaking to the driver they discovered this was because he had to pick up more nurses, as some night shift nurses had telephoned to say they would not be reporting for duty. The hospital authorities thus thought it appropriate to ask the nurses in the morning shift to replace the absent night shift nurses. The nurses told me that this was not uncommon. Even when they are tired, they go thinking of the patients who need their services. Overtime duty was not paid earlier but was introduced in many hospitals from 2005, though not in the small nursing homes. Thus, these hostels provided by hospitals ensure a 'backup' of nurses to run the system. It is no secret that the nurse-patient ratios are well below the standard 1:6 and are even 1:35 or 1:50 in private hospitals.

Nevertheless, nurses think that it is safer to have the hospital ambulance pick them up rather than depend on other forms of transport like rickshaws for short distances, or walking. They also consider hostel accommodation as more acceptable for their parents and family in Kerala.

Those who rented houses did so because they wanted more privacy. Some did so when they wanted family members to come and stay with them. A few could not adjust to the timings for their coaching and study for the IELTS and CGFNS, and so opted to rent houses outside. There were a few who chose, from the very beginning, to stay with friends because they found it economical. Some just continued living with the friends through whom they had obtained their jobs. Whatever the reasons for their living arrangement, they all seem to have two preferences—the roommate/house mate had to be a Malayali and a nurse.

> It helps to have a Malayali as roommate. You can cook the same meal and there are no adjustment issues. Nurses understand the problems of night shifts and ... will not mind the change in schedule and sleep(ing) during the daytime. Others find it difficult. We prefer nurses as housemates...

Marie, for example, stays in the hostel because her husband is working as a foreman in Abu Dhabi. She was not amenable to sharing her possible migration plans with me and was therefore careful so as to not reveal anything unintentionally. But she was interested in the migration of nurses to various places and finally admitted that she wanted to live with her husband in the Gulf or even in Europe or America. Her husband had departed after one month of their marriage and she had continued to stay in the hostel. Her pattern of life did not change with marriage, except that she now calls her in-laws several times a month along with the calls she makes to her parents in Kerala.

Sheeba says that she settled in Delhi after her marriage to a Delhi boy, a businessman. She had no migration plans at the time of the interview, although she had spent some time in the Gulf working as a staff nurse. She says she earned a good salary in Saudi Arabia and used to send the money to her parents who, in turn, spent it on her marriage. Sheeba was clear in that even if she did migrate she would not really like to return to the Gulf because as a Christian she did not have the freedom to practise her faith there. She rates the life of a nurse in the Gulf as superior to life in Delhi in only one respect: technological superiority due to advanced equipment for patient care in hospitals. Social life is a zero, she said.

> They have money... and working in those hospitals, you really feel good, not like our hospitals that are overcrowded...[with] outdated machines. But here I enjoy the social life. I do not even want

to settle in Kerala. I prefer Delhi...Kerala is also very expensive...It is [good] for visiting relatives once a while, not too often though [laughs...].[15]

For every successful story and for every helping hand for the present crop of migrant nurses, there are untold stories of those who migrated first, of those already in the new city, who now must host the new migrants. These are the women who have described their experience as 'the heat of migration', which the present generation does not face. They felt disadvantaged that there was no one to protect them in their time and inform them of the tribulations they would face in Delhi. This often surfaces when they believe that they have some grievance against the larger family. Bincy, who did her BSc in Nursing, does not want to join military nursing and also does not want to continue in an Indian hospital. She says that it was very difficult to get admission in the degree course and this is surely the opportunity for her to improve her standard of life. She was born in Kerala but did her schooling in Delhi. As a result she never felt 'the heat of migration'. But she witnessed her cousins from Kerala having to struggle while hunting for a job here. She realised from what she had seen that starting life in a strange place is very hard on women. Her family hosted many uncles, aunts and cousins who came to Delhi in search of jobs. Her father's sister's daughter was the last one to complete her GNM from Karnataka and was (at the time of the interview) working as a staff nurse in Apollo Hospital. In spite of being sympathetic to the difficulties of migrants, Bincy discovered that there were problems to face while hosting migrants from Kerala. Being guests, high standards of treatment are expected; this can be difficult for an urban family due to lack of space and other constraints. Sometimes relations do become strained because of the high expectations of the guests. This is something that I am familiar with. As a child whose family was staying in the cantonment in Mumbai, I have vivid memories of my mother complaining about my father's relatives—men coming to stay in search of jobs.

Delhi Hospitals as Workplaces

In its annual report for the year 2005–6 the Comptroller and Auditor General of India says that hospitals in Delhi are deficient

in many areas.[16] Shortage of ambulance services or the sheer
lack of essential medicines and equipment are highlighted in
the report. Four major hospitals account for 32 per cent of the
total bed strength in the public hospitals in the capital—Lok
Nayak, Deen Dayal Upadhyay, Charak Palika and Hindurao.
Of these, three could not make available 19–26 per cent of the
essential medicines to terminally ill patients. Procurement,
installation and commissioning of equipment involve a lot of
corruption and delay in 72 per cent of the cases. A severe shortage of nursing and other medical and paramedical staff is reported. Ambulances are misused; more than 50 per cent of
ambulance use is not for patients. Of the four hospitals, two
of them—Charak Palika and Lok Nayak—did not have basic
life support equipment. Waste disposal is far below standard.
Storage, management and disposal of this waste are not in
keeping with the Biomedical Waste Storage, Management and
Disposal Rules of 1998. This is the state of the general safety
of our hospitals, and as workplaces they pose a serious health
hazard to the nurses, apart from patients and general public.

There are significant variations in the technical qualifications, appearance, meanings and terms of competence and efficiency of the nurses across the types of hospitals that I visited.
Service conditions and salary also vary according to institutions. While super-speciality hospitals and government hospitals
assure permanent employment, small and medium enterprises
do not guarantee such permanency. Permanency is accompanied
by the right to avail leave and other benefits approved by the
government, including the basic right of maternity leave. In
small nursing homes, duties are not clearly defined and there
is no written agreement between the employer and the nurses.
Consequently, nurses end up doing both skilled and unskilled
jobs in the wards, as well as various administrative functions.
Usha, whom I first mistook to be a receptionist, tells me:

> Yes, I attend to phone calls because there is no receptionist.
> There are doctors who visit [the nursing home] for fixed hours,
> unless there is some emergency. They are available [in case of
> emergency only] for twenty-four hours a day on call. But nurses
> are here all the time. Some of the nurses stay on the top floor of
> the nursing home...We fill up the register and go with doctors for
> routine ward duty in the morning... there are these two men for

help (with the patients). They go out in case we need to buy some things. They do other types of jobs like lifting male patients and moving beds and so on...

Those migrating from Kerala—for reasons as varied as high unemployment rates, poor working conditions in the hospitals and nursing homes, a desire to travel and see the world, learn new languages and, most importantly, to earn their living and become self-reliant—do not, therefore, find their hopes answered in Delhi. Working in Delhi hospitals has not been a very enjoyable experience for many of my respondents; it is more a stepping stone to better things.

For the young and unmarried, and for some married women, there is a clear purpose in their stay in Delhi—it is part of a larger plan. My study found a distinct difference in the attitude of young nurses (22–30 years) and their older counterparts. Young nurses clearly treat their stay in Delhi as short-term, as part of the strategy to migrate to greener pastures. Everyone in this group is preparing for or has already passed the IELTS and CGFNS. Some are taking a longer route through the Persian Gulf and have appeared for interviews for employment in hospitals there.[17] For the older nurses, migration is not their most important plan at present because they cannot be 'footloose' like single women. Family migration, nevertheless, is explored as a possibility, but moving from Delhi requires a lot of preparation and upsets the rhythm of their present lives. In practical terms, they find it difficult to disturb the schooling of their children and the hard-earned comfort in Delhi.

Differences in the degree of comfort at their respective workplaces, places of residence and differences in work culture and professionalism are evident. There are differences in the contractual nature of the job in various hospitals and in the notion of permanence between the government sector, large private hospitals and smaller nursing homes. The nursing sector in Delhi offers an interesting example of the mixture of organised and unorganised sectors, of regulation and chaos. Many in the private sector do not follow any regulations regarding leave packages. Maternity leave is not allowed—the moment a nurse reports her pregnancy, she can be asked to leave.

Malayali nurses have been employed in large numbers in Delhi hospitals for many decades now. Old and young nurses

speak about their numerous disabilities and handicaps as women
nurses and as 'outsiders' in Delhi. These include issues like the
lack of a proper place to stay, the status of nurses/nursing, and
their poor working conditions. However, there did not seem to
be any effort towards a collective agency to redress such grievances or to at least protest about their unsatisfactory work
conditions.

Among hospitals that do not follow any regulations (whatever they might profess on paper in order to register with the
Delhi health department), some operate with the owner or the
manager as the norm, with all rules and regulations rolled into
one person. In short, he is the 'god' who cannot be brought to
book because he is the ultimate authority and has perceptible
political connections.

(a) **Issues of Minimum Wages**: Most private hospitals in Delhi
flout the norms regarding minimum wages. There are
reported to be discrepancies in the accounts maintained
by many hospitals for audit purposes as far as the wages
of nurses are concerned. Actual amounts paid and the salaries mentioned in the register differ in nursing homes
that pay their employees in cash. Under-qualified, B-grade
nurses are employed in place of A-grade nurses, resulting
in a situation where nurses collude with the management
to flout the norms on qualifications.

From not paying minimum wages to the ruthless treatment of nurses as servants are two ends of a continuum.
The same management running two different hospitals—
one private and the other charitable—is not uncommon
either. In such cases, the treatment of nurses differs. In
the charitable trust, nurses are paid below the minimum
wage in cash by the manager and they do not sign any
documents. One register is kept for this purpose but is not
official. In other nursing homes, a register with a higher
amount as paid salary is reported to exist.

(b) **Lack of Monitoring:** There is no regular examination or
inspection of the hospitals by the health department.
Though the Directorate of Health of the Delhi government
has stipulated requirements for the registration of nursing
homes, it is hardly followed and there is no periodic

inspection to check whether the nursing homes follow the regulations.

(c) **Lack of Adherence to Rules:** This extends to not giving the stipulated legal entitlements to individual nurses. In many small hospitals there is no maternity leave or benefits for the nurses. Often, hospitals cannot be sued because nurses collude with the authorities. In some cases there are no proper documents to prove malpractices in a court of law. For example, Jalaja was working as a staff nurse in Sunderlal Jain Hospital and had her second child. She had to 'resign' (in other words, asked to leave) because the hospital had no provision for maternity leave in the hospital.

> I worked in another hospital before my job in Sunderlal Jain ... the salary was not good and then after five years I joined this place [Sunderlal Jain]. The salary was better and so was the work. Moreover I could walk to the hospital from my home. ... Now they asked me to leave when I became pregnant. But I also left my job when I was pregnant with the older child (while working in the other hospital).

Jalaja does not consider it an offence that the hospital asked her to leave when she became pregnant. She claimed that there are no provisions for maternity leave and so she could not have done anything about it. Her response is probably calculated in terms of the fact that she had no certificate to prove her eligibility to work as a staff nurse. In any case, the hospital would not have wanted to risk a problem by employing a pregnant woman. What is significant for our study is that due to the shortage of nurses and unorganised nature of nursing work in the private sector, hospital authorities are able to exploit the labour of both skilled nurses and underqualified women who work as nurses.

Jalaja, despite her struggles in Delhi, has been able to find some sources of social support from the local community. She is happy to be staying where she is because the landlady who is active in the women's organisation—Janawadi Mahila Samiti—is very kind-hearted and helps

with the older child. She is also lenient with rent pay-
ments. The household has the bare minimum in terms of
furniture, making the financial hardship actually visible,
possibly exacerbated by additional guests from Kerala.

(d) **Unregulated Privatisation:** The years of economic liberalisation have entered the health sector as well. Delhi
has a fairly large health care sector promoted by private
entrepreneurs and this largely segregated health care
market in the city has now become even more unregulated. Measures that help the processes of privatisation
and worsen working conditions are deepening in the
name of professionalism and competition. Nurses face a
particularly difficult situation, though this is not unique
to India. Everywhere, including in the US, nurses bear the
brunt of cost cutting. One can observe double standards
in two areas—wages and flexibility. The wages of nurses
remain more or less constant, while doctors (called consultants) get handsome fees and better terms of work.
While flexibility is the buzzword for doctors, nurses are
asked to sign contracts for a minimum of two years. Thus,
the terms and conditions by which hospitals make sure
that doctors and nurses are retained differ. While doctors
are not bound by commitment to the hospital after duty
hours, nurses are restricted from applying elsewhere by
their contracts.[18] It has been found that the 'proportion of
wages paid to consultants has shot up in recent years; for
instance, doctors in large private hospitals currently earn
five times the salary of their counterparts in the All India
Institute of Medical Sciences' (AIIMS) (Workers' Solidarity
Report 2000: 4). Globalisation and privatisation processes
in the health care sector in India are associated, by their
promoters, with international standards of infrastructure,
efficiency and quality care. Steps taken in this direction
are visible in the form of tall, glass buildings and contract labourers, making it possible to select young and
dynamic people as workers. In large corporate hospitals,
the paramedical and ancillary levels of staff have been
contracted to outside agencies to control labour costs.
They include ward boys, security guards, sweepers and
so on.

This arrangement leads to a lack of camaraderie and even interaction between various levels of workers. The contractors' relationship with individual workers is one of total dependency and control. Norms regarding both minimum wages and number of hours of work are flouted in private hospitals (ibid.). Any possibility of a platform for collective action is prevented, as the terms of[19] employment do not allow any interaction among workers or between workers and their de facto employers.

The policy of hiring contract labour has an adverse effect on the unionisation of workers. As such, nurses are among the least organised workers—collective bargaining is not feasible even in premier institutions like AIIMS due to management hostility and the adverse attitudes of higher authorities.[20] All laws regarding minimum wages and service conditions are contravened. The monthly earnings of the paramedical and ancillary staff of the private hospitals is much lower than in state-owned hospitals (Baru 2004). Minimum wages are not paid in most of the small nursing homes, which are registered with the Delhi local administration. Poor terms of employment, low standards of work, poor living conditions and poor quality of training characterise the paramedical and support staff. 'Casualisation' of labour and selective international labour mobility are additional issues.

(e) **Hierarchy within the Hospital:** The hospital hierarchy gives prime importance to the physicians, while nurses are generally seen as subordinates who assist them in patient care. Nurses are placed under the medical fraternity administratively and are under the direct supervision of the medical officer in a hospital.

Nurses complain that doctors and patients often underestimate the role of nurses in patient care. Ignorance about the education and skills of the nurses also leads to mistreatment of nurses in public. Some doctors even shout at them, forgetting that nurses are complementary to doctors in the system of patient care.

(f) **Hierarchy within Nursing:** In the small private hospitals registered with the Delhi local administration, minimum wages are not paid to nurses who are often underqualified and sometimes unqualified. In the case of these 'B-grade' nurses who have received training in ANM, their chances of going abroad are also lower than those of 'A-grade' nurses who have a diploma or a degree in nursing and midwifery.

The exploitation of nurses, as the nurses' union would put it, is a serious issue and contributes to their international migration, mainly for better service conditions and status. Nonetheless, there is another dimension to the unregulated nature of the health sector, namely, the large number of unqualified women who practise as nurses. The combination of such a situation, together with ignorance of legal norms, lack of support mechanisms, and lack of fluency in the local language are reasons why many nurses do not come out to protest.

Pushpa, who never received a certificate for her ANM training, was taught to give injections to patients at her job and, according to her, the regular patients prefer her for the job to the other nurses in her nursing home.

> I did my ANM course in a private institute...and went to practise [as part of the course] in a well-known hospital nearby. I learnt everything well; they [teachers] were good... But by the time we were to get our certificate, that centre closed down because the government refused to recognise that place... We (our batch) did not get any certificate...those before us—our seniors—who got the (provisional) certificate from the institute saying that they did this course from the institute and the recognition was applied for, etc., they had no use with their certificates. There were lab technicians, pharmacy students. Then I had no money to do any course... I was preparing to come to Delhi with a friend when I got married to someone who works in Delhi and from then on started working here. I get ₹2,500 every month. When I started I was getting ₹1,000...

When I interviewed Pushpa, she was hoping to use the experience of working as a nurse in this nursing home elsewhere on better terms, which often only means a marginal increase in salary.[21]

If we look around, we see migrant men and women who work in other areas and professions following similar trajectories to those of nurses. So what is so special about these nurses whose experiences I have detailed here? Other than the fact that nurses form the single largest category of educated women migrating for work, there is nothing unique or extraordinary about them. And yet it is this very ordinariness of these migrant women, as they negotiate the most daunting socio-economic structures and norms of the family on an everyday basis, that makes them so interesting.

Whether it is their wages, working conditions or living conditions, there are no clear policies or satisfactory implementation of existing rules. This is partly due to Delhi's health sector, which has the characteristics of both the unorganised and organised sectors. The status of their profession and their gender are played out in the socio-cultural and geographical space of Delhi, which almost never becomes a permanent place of residence. Their hopes and plans are about 'moving elsewhere' while their roots and structures of existence are in various villages and towns of Kerala.

Therefore, it is often said that nurse migrants from Kerala do not mind moving to another city or to another country because it makes no difference to them where they stay. But how can this be true? Obviously nurses do not think so. Their decisions to move are complex and heterogeneous, though all the outsider sees is a homogeneous entity, namely, 'the migrant Malayali nurse'. The next chapter looks more closely at the lives of nurses as migrants in Delhi; it describes how each nurse has a unique understanding of her situation and that is what shapes her aspirations, needs and experiences. The dense identities of being a woman, nurse and Malayali operate simultaneously and sometimes separately, but usually in a complex combination, depending on circumstances.

Notes

1. Harzig (2001), in her historical analysis, explains how as a member of larger migration systems and more specific sub systems, a 'femina migrans' makes use of 'a goodly portion of agency' that is instilled in her.

2. Many studies on migrant women in India are anxious about physical safety and this is reflected in the responses of the respondents. Sexual harassment and molestation are primary

concerns and the association is more with the honour of women than their physical safety.

3. One exception is Kavya (28 years old) who was employed in an SEZ and never got any training in nursing but was directly employed as a nurse in a 15-bed hospital in north-west Delhi where her sister, who is an ANM, has been employed. This case is very different from the rest of the nurses who have some sort of training, but migrants who are unskilled (and even skilled) get exploited at various stages of their migration.

4. According to a rough estimate. See *Mathrubhoomi*, 28 November 2009, p. 10.

5. It is curious that Morrison did not spot even a single nurse among 'the secondary school graduates of the 1960s and 1970s' who, he reported, were engineers, doctors, teachers and research scientists, despite his empathetic research on the marginalised in Kerala society.

6. The five volumes on women and migration in Asia brought out by Developing Countries Research Centre (2003) and published by Sage Publications have a large number of micro studies that fascinate us with the stories of different types of migration—workseeking, marriage and displacement-induced—that rely heavily on networking and connections.

7. Implementation of the Sixth Pay Commission during 2009–10 is reported to have influenced nurses in their decision to stay on in Indian hospitals. Nurses say that opportunities to go to countries like the UK have also shrunk.

8. For IELTS and CGFNS.

9. Malayalis, in general, are perceived as an ethnic group with high levels of solidarity and networking by others, as mentioned earlier.

10. The authors do critique the social capital model for the lack of consideration it has for the ways in which gender inequality structures social capital by following the line of argument by Mayoux (2001).

11. It is assumed that you are 'naturally' part of the 'group if you are a nurse from Kerala. If one tries to be close to other nurses who are from Delhi and tries to keep only professional contact with Malayali nurses, she is described with phrases like a 'show-off' or someone trying to act smart, which have negative connotations. These nurses are eventually treated as outcasts.

12. One interesting case is that of M. Kumar in Delhi who explained how his life in Delhi as a migrant was miserable during the first year of his arrival when his mother, younger brother and sister expected him to send a large amount of money for them every

month. And this was when he, as a typist, was finding it difficult to survive due to a low salary and language problems. He could not speak English or Hindi fluently and finally left Delhi for his village on a local ticket as he did not even have money to reserve his ticket after a bout of severe viral fever. When he reached home, he could not tell his real story to his family because of the prevailing image of him as coming back home for a vacation. Within a week he had returned to Delhi after a phone conversation with a friend and had decided to try and make it in Delhi. This was because he decided to not be a failure in front of the villagers. I am indebted to Mr Kumar for his story and his opinion on the community's insensitivity towards an individual who is lost in the migration flow. His illustrations on moments of contrasting emotions at the time of his failed migration and his subsequent success story as a valued manager in a travel agency are invaluable.

13. *Ulvili* in Malayalam.
14. A few nurses in my sample lived in private hostels in the neighbourhood, aimed primarily at working migrant women from outside the city. Practices here regarding the movement of nurses remain more or less the same though there seemed to be fewer restrictions in terms of timings. Moreover, not all the women are nurses.
15. This opinion is shared by many like Anusha, Mridula and Shijy.
16. As reported in the *Times of India*, 21 April 2007.
17. When continuing with my interviews in Shanti Mukand, four of my respondents reported having been selected for hospitals in Kuwait. The same was the case with Maharaja Agrasen Hospital where the nurses did not even inform the management about their plans to leave nor did they collect their security cash deposit from the hospital.
18. Apollo Hospital claims to facilitate the migration of its staff to western countries by opening study centres for IELTS within the hospital complex. In fact, this provides even stricter control over their movements.
19. Often, strict implementation of norms that are not part of formal terms of employment also prevents nurses from sharing their grievances that may lead to collective action. Some hospitals sanction nurses from speaking among themselves in their mother tongue and this is a strategy to discourage these women from creating groups within hospitals. Speaking in languages that the patients are not familiar with, especially languages other than Hindi and English, is alleged to create an uncomfortable ambience for patients.

20. Vanitha (34 years old), for example, says that many of the high-profile doctors in AIIMS are against nurses claiming any more rights than what has been given. She also agrees that being a public sector organisation, AIIMS provides nurses with all possible facilities but the attitude of doctors towards nurses is often pathetic.
21. Pushpa stopped working in 2008 as her husband felt she was failing in her duties at home. At the time she was getting ₹3,500 per month.

5

Reconstructing Identities
Diasporic Politics and Gender in Delhi

This chapter[1] looks at the main ways in which migrant women nurses are (re)figured in the diasporic conditions of Delhi. Malayalis do not form a diaspora in any conventional sense, but there is 'a dispersion of a people, language, or culture that was formerly concentrated in one place'; Kerala, in a certain sense, is also 'the Promised Land' for there is hope that they will return, a nostalgia that is heartbreaking. Diaspora here is used in a more metaphorical sense, indicating the deeper connection between a locale, its culture and the different forms of identification people prefer when they are away from 'home'. This longing to be 'home' is split from the experiences of a Kerala that has failed them. Stark experiences of the 'educated population that is un-employed' in Kerala and opinions like the following are heard often: 'Nothing interesting happens in Kerala; people gossip a lot and interfere in others' lives'. Nevertheless, their identities in Delhi are reconstructed through selective reminiscences of the Kerala they have left behind. Romanticisation and construc-tions of a perfect past are entrenched in the Malayali con-sciousness, epitomised by the Keralam ruled by Mahabali, the *asura* King.

> *Maveli Naadu vanidum kalam*
> *Manusharellarumonnupole*
> *Kallavum Illa Chathium Illa*
> *Kallatharangal Mattonnumilla*[2]

Malayali identity (like others') is fluid and changing despite the insistence on originality and authenticity. The very authenticity of the culture is also imagined and created along the way. There are also claims to a genuine Malayali-ness unavailable in Kerala, like the Joint Secretary of the Dwarka Malayalee Association who says: '...There is no Onam in Kerala... It is we — who are outside Kerala — who celebrate these festivals with sincerity and dedication...as it should be (celebrated).'

This discourse divulges the deep need of migrant Malayalis for an authentic Kerala, which acts as a reference point on more than one occasion. Being migrants, their personal, professional and social lives are sensitive to the volatility of the ideologies of the state, religion and larger society. They form an ethnic and linguistic minority group in the community-led identity politics of the Indian capital. As elsewhere, Malayali identity in Delhi is constructed through male migrants, despite the fact that the migration of Malayali nurses is as old as those of the men. Yet discussion ignores the distinct identity and visibility of 'Malayali nurses'. In that sense it goes beyond 'invisibilising' the nurse; rather, it maligns the single woman migrant typified by her. The single woman migrant personified by the nurse is made to stand out from others due to her perceived freedom. This image does not fit with notions of ideal Malayali womanhood[3] and bring enormous discomfort to the 'pure' Malayali patriarchal notions[4] and disrepute to the 'chaste' Malayali woman. This woman is 'protected' on all sides, by father, mother, brothers, neighbours and even fellow villagers through their chaperoning 'stare'. Needless to say, the average Malayali woman should not be left alone, which is why she has to look down when she walks, being uncomfortable with the 'gaze' that follows her.

Rani tells me that she preferred to stay with her grandparents near Ernakulam city rather than at her parents' place in rural Idukki district. She recounts her unease in encountering on a daily basis the stares of the men of the village while they sat at the bus stop. She finally complained to her parents that she could no longer endure it. Her parents understood the problem and asked her grandparents to accommodate her.[5] Clearly, in her mind, the relative anonymity of a city like Ernakulam compared to the claustrophobic and closed atmosphere offers a freer public space to women.

Being a Malayali has been strongly shaped by the claim of being more 'socially developed' than the rest of India, to the point of superiority over fellow Indians. This claim of a higher cultural existence and exceptionalism has been supported by development indicators of high literacy, good primary health care and low infant mortality rates and even 'good cinema', this being defined as realistic cinema that transcends the 'supposed' divide between art and mainstream cinema and has a distinct identity (Osella and Osella 2006: 173).[6] The low per capita income of Kerala made these achievements look extraordinary.[7] It is indisputable that the social equality inherent in Marxist ideology did help Kerala after the first communist regime took over in 1957. Social welfare measures, the land ceiling act, and relatively better access to modern education raised standards to a level comparable to many developed societies of the north, in spite of very low economic advancement even in relation to other Indian states. Nevertheless, entrenched social hierarchies based on caste and gender never disappeared from the social terrain of Kerala; rather, they were created and made visible in the consciousness of common people through complex histories of social reform.

In recent times, many critiques busted the highly misguided notion of Kerala women's high status in society, especially with reports on the abominable level of violence against women in domestic and public spaces (Mukhopadhyay 2007). In fact, there has been 'rising visibility of gender-based violence, particularly domestic violence, mental illness manifested increasingly as suicide, and the rapid growth and spread of dowry and related crimes' (Eapen and Kodoth 2003: 228). The gender insensitivity of the major political parties is demonstrable in the low number of women as peoples' representatives in the state and central assemblies. Political parties put up an abysmally small number of candidates from this gender in their panels. For a decade or two, Malayali exceptionalism—the image of Kerala as a progressive society that is so different than the rest of India—worked to invisibilise the forms of patriarchy that seemed to be mediating women's and men's lives in Kerala. This institutionalisation of complex forms of patriarchal power has not been sufficiently noted in the academic discourse which gave all its attention to 'higher' political consciousness, social awareness and levels of education. All varieties of reformist discourse during colonialism and after—the colonial officials, the missionaries, the English-educated Malayalis, even that of the left intellectuals—drew upon a strident opposition between 'progress' and 'ignorance/superstition', and the faith that the latter would be overcome by rooting out its material, social and ideological conditions of existence. On the other hand, the reality of women's status in Kerala included a disproportionately large share of the burden of contraception and sexual morality on women, especially of the educated middle class of Malayali society (Devika 2005: 345–46) and the responsibility for domestic violence on themselves.

Otherwise different, if not conflicted institutions such as the left, the church and other groups that emerged in civil society have grounded their conceptions of modernity and development in the notion of the sacramental nuclear and reproductive family. As the basis of the Malayali sense of social well being, it is no wonder that the 'proper management' of women's sexuality becomes a matter of community concern.[8] As Devika points out in this discussion, even the family planning agenda had to bring in this family image to keep itself going.

The massive discourse of the Kerala model also blurred the changing forms of oppression within society that were unquestioned. It is within these contexts that we must locate and deconstruct the image of the Malayali nurse—'daring' if not 'empowered', capable of working 'alone' in any context, anywhere in the world. Yet she is very much the product of Kerala's agrarian crisis, expected to serve her family, always apologetic for having been born as a girl, having to migrate to earn a living and earn her own dowry, and then be at the receiving end of moral judgements on her character.

Malayalis and Others

Kerala, 'God's Own Country', exists in the minds of the '*pravasis*' or diaspora as 'home'. They belong to that Kerala and Kerala belongs to them. Here, as Anderson (1983) puts it, ethnic nationalism of the sort demonstrated by Malayalis is fashioned into existence as an imagined community. These imaginations are constituted by tales of local temple '*utsavam*' or church '*perunnal*'[9] and how as adolescents and later as young men, they used to spend their time with friends in the festival grounds. And, yes, this is the stuff of nostalgia that Kerala men are made of, differing substantially from the way women think of their past lives. While men's reminiscences about their enjoyment are about public spaces beyond the domestic, for women it is primarily the domestic: how they cooked a dish for the first time, or about the collective called the family and its controlling freedom even in public spaces. Or, again, how all the children from the extended family used to meet during Onam, Christmas and so on, thus cementing the 'domestic' as the most important component of nostalgia.

It would be wrong, however, to completely deny the possibility of the domestic in the minds of men but it is a space which they can renounce when they want to and emerge into the public. It seems like they project what they are expected to, maybe unconsciously; that their 'legitimate' concern is over the public space rather than private and domestic. Moreover, it is shrouded in a surreal existence, dreamlike and carpeted by the wellness and goodness of the family! Occasionally one hears memories filled with the pangs of poverty and symbols of alienation. And yet the marshmallow of indigenous myths, in my reading of it, is able to combine with modernist elements. Political, social and historical imaginations co-exist in a complex manner to make it the kind of imagination that is anti-colonial and self-sufficient in the way that Chatterjee (1994a: 6) has described it. And its middle-class attitude is shaped not by rejection of modernity but a selection from among the many, quite in line with the nationalists discussed by Chatterjee (1994b).

They look at the 'wider Malayali community' as their own and envision a greater Kerala which extends in a social space beyond the physical space of Kerala, the narrow strip stretching from *mala* (the hills) till *ala* (the waves), thus forming the physical space of Malayalam. To quote from Marie Percot:

> In an average Malayali family there will be a brother in Saudi Arabia, another one in Dubai, a sister in Kuwait, an uncle in Canada, an aunt in U.K. and maybe some cousins in the States or Australia... So we Malayalis feel a little bit as if the world was ours and that Kerala was only the centre of it... (2006: 162).

> ...see here for example, wherever you go you meet a Malayali... in the markets, in the buses, in the church... And my eyes are well-trained in recognising Malayalis in the streets... that when you were standing at the reception I saw you and thought ...oh this one looks like one Malayali... And see you are one... (Annamma)

In this study, I have not focussed on the legal aspects of relocation, citizenship and domicile status in Delhi. However, citizenship issues do arise because of the 'difference' the nurses bring with them to the new locale. And as I have brought out in an article on rethinking citizenship, the modern notion of citizenship is mediated by gender, linguistic and ethnic identities (Nair 2007: 137–56). And their right to the space of Delhi as workers gives them formal grounds that arbitrate their experience of Indian citizenship. This difference is visualised and articulated vis-à-vis the 'others', the local population and other migrants who, despite their heterogeneous origins, are referred to as 'north Indians' by the nurses.

Malayali identity (like other identities) also takes shape in its contrast with others; it is, therefore, others who help define Malayali identity in their diasporic setting. Similarly, identity politics within the Malayali community creates and isolates a monolith called 'the nurse'. This woman is different from other Malayali women because she is a nurse; she is morally corrupt and gullible, since she is not visibly under the control of the community.

At one level, existing gender norms are being rejected and yet at another level are being reconstructed. Thus, as discussed by Boyd and Grieco (2003: 2–3),

> ...the content of gender—what constitutes the ideals, expectations, and behaviors or expressions of masculinity and femininity — will vary among societies. Also, when people interact with each other, by adhering to this content or departing from it, they either reaffirm or change what is meant by gender, thus affecting social relationships at a particular time or in a particular setting.

As George argues, 'at both individual and social levels, this new female earning power was undefined and unnegotiated' (2005: 44). Questioning the possession of these women—their economic resources and sexuality—at some level is at the root of this reconstruction.

Nurses and others

Identity politics within the migrant Malayali community is composed of various dimensions based on caste, class, gender, family status and place of origin back in Kerala. Here it is the 'nurse' as a category vis-à-vis the other groups that is being explored. George (2000, 2005) has discussed the differentiated existence of nurses and their families in the context of Malayali Christian migrants in a US city in relation to their counterparts in other occupations. Nurses are identified as of 'low' class origins and hence any ties with their families are disapproved of. They are 'dirty' (George 2000); husbands are, relatively speaking, unwelcome in an otherwise noble gathering of Malayali migrants precisely because initiative and agency has been taken by women to reach the land where 'milk and honey flow'. The coarseness of these attitudes is masked in the subtlety of gender politics in which these nurses and their husbands also play into the 'patriarchal bargain'[10] that is highly entrenched in notions of class difference and status.

Another important discussion concerns the relation between nurses and other women among the Malayali migrants. There are two kinds of responses—formal and informal—about nurses from other women. One is replete with scandal and stories of adventure. These stories have their variations and add-ons. A left activist who later went on to become an important national-level office bearer of a women's organisation constructed the image of an improbable 'typical' young Malayali nurse in Delhi in the following manner. According to her, the young nurse went on to have at least five illegal abortions in clinics in the nearby satellite city of Faridabad. The heart of the narrative revolves around the nurse's single status and the absence of a male family figure.

And what about the Malayali men? They, like Mohanan Pillai[11] below, acquaint others around them with stories of nurses doubling up as sex workers.

> ...Oh! Let me tell you about nurses, I have seen with my eyes, how they sit on cots outside their rooms in Govindpuri area ...soliciting customers... with the result that every Malayali woman here gets a bad name... They do everything that is not in our *samskaram* (culture)... I also know a story ... not a story but a real incident where the nurse jumped off the wall of the working women's hostel...at night...I do not have to describe her character...These things are happening...You just have to try... they are ready to come with you...

The question of how he thought only nurses did what they were alleged to be doing was evaded and I was told that nurses were notorious for their 'boldness'. What is clear is that sexual fantasies have fastened onto nurses who are already stereotyped.

This portrayal has the further function of maintaining the sanctity of others who, 'like us—me and my wife and sister' are clean and pure. 'Our *samskaram*' was defined as being modest, keeping away from strange men, not being found alone in a public space and being obedient. Who, then, is the ideal Malayali woman migrant? To many the stereotype of a good Malayali woman migrant is a housewife married to a Malayali man owning a car and has two children, who can at most aspire to be a school teacher. Though I do not venture into that, one can identify a class character of the Malayali migrants' patriarchy. Various dilemmas and equations among women migrants on issues like earnings and standards of living are played out around questions of sexuality, by creating nurses in the image of the prostitute.

While sharing the dilemmas of the migrant Malayalis, not much distinction was made by the nurses of the study between the local Hindi speaking population and non-Malayali migrant people. The latter categories were clubbed together as others who came into the discussion as and when they got some direct personal and professional interaction. Some references to the possible migrant status of others with whom they interact on an everyday basis came up mainly in the stories of Sindhu, Diana and some other respondents where the former were recognisable as patients, competing colleagues, neighbours, and those who were met within a public space. As narrated by Sindhu, nurses see themselves as being perceived as 'poor women' who need to work but at the same time this opinion seems to vary across class categories and seems to be changing as well. Though shortage of nurses has not done much to change this perception, migration opportunities seem to be contributing towards the change that is still not widespread. Anyhow these women are seen as competing with the rest of the population in Delhi for space and resources that might have resulted in experiences like that of Diana or lead to comments from the local population like that by Monica (quoted in the section below). Interviews also revealed that nurses imbibe the images and opinions floating around and think, like Rani, that the bad reputation of the nurses is due to the flow in the character of 'some' nurses. These narrations are few and difficult to be put together as data and yet form important sources of information, for this is how the everyday experiences are shaped in reality.

Thus, nurses appear as stereotypes of a particular lifestyle and as loose women who are ready to sell themselves for easy money, despite the fact that they have one of the hardest jobs in Delhi. The sexual stereotyping of nurses is also a strategy to make sense of new systems of power relations in a space where single women without their families are making a living. This breaks the traditional understanding of dependent gender relations. Reading between the lines, nurses, due to their social and economic disadvantages, are stereotyped in ways that explain and justify the disparities back home. The fact that Malayalis keep a distance from the nurses whom they see only in hospitals adds to the convoluted perception and stigmatisation.

Hoffman and Hurst (1990), who have worked on gender stereotypes, believe that they arise from the need to explain and justify people's activities and social roles. Stereotypes do not necessarily represent realities but do help explain the power equation in a group or locale. Groups which have disadvantaged positions in the traditional social and economic hierarchy are often at the receiving end of such stereotyping. Thus, the stereotyping of Malayali nurses does not exist in isolation; rather, it is tied to the entire organisation of Malayali social life in Delhi and the transfer of traditional hierarchies from Kerala to Delhi. Attributing a loose sexual morality to nurses provides order to changing gender equations. The anomaly of single, earning women, their economic power and their rather free movement are feared and this situation that is new and different results in internal othering in order to shore up the 'mainstream' Malayali.

This stereotyping, therefore, directly defines mainstream 'Malayali-ness' in Delhi, where the nurse is the other and where a Malayali woman is everything that a nurse is not. Patricia Devine (1989: 7) has argued that categorisation and association are two fundamental concepts involved in stereotyping. This can happen outside our explicit awareness. When we create a stereotype, we usually make a list of traits that go together and are associated with particular groups of people. Thus, Malayali nurses are 'daring women who are in search of some easy money through any means'. They have identifiable characteristics as women who work at night and with strange men. They also pollute themselves by dealing in bodily fluids like urine and blood. Those who stereotype try to bring to mind examples of stereotyped people and the behaviours associated with the stereotype.

At the same time, remarks by the non-Malayali population such as 'nurses have spoiled your (Malayali women's) name in Delhi' bring out the wider dynamic that reinforces the distancing by non-nurses. The unconscious use of some stereotypes embarrasses the users and the listener to a great extent as both see more and more nurses around them in their everyday lives. However, stereotypes can change and this has happened with nurses too. The sacred veil of respectability, according to many older nurses, is slowly embracing the nursing community. Material factors of better salary and working conditions are reported as reasons.

It is clear from the narrations of nurses that recreation of the cultural and social context of Kerala with its hierarchies and control mechanisms is attempted in Delhi and yet, as Shijy and Rani spelt out clearly, this is less constraining than that of Kerala. In Delhi nurses are able to exercise their agency as individuals beyond the family space which Shijy is so happy to leave behind. Moreover, they have access to the formal rights of workers however inadequate these rights are. Not a single nurse thought of Delhi as more oppressive than Kerala and all of them were unanimous that financial independence does provide women with choices.

Sites of Identity Politics

The identity politics of the migrants in our study is not staged as any singular acting but as part of everyday life, giving it a mundane aura. Its profanity is reduced in its effect, making it 'normal', everyday practice. Most Malayalis in Delhi are steeped in interactions within the Malayali community, and sometimes limited by it, with the result that even after years of staying in Delhi they are not equipped to deal fluently in Hindi or in English. Malayali families become familiar and friendly with another Malayali family living in the next neighbourhood or colony much more than the non-Malayali family staying right next door.[12]

This is an important aspect of the blame game that goes on between the migrants and the locals as to who has to be more responsible for the integration process, reminding one of the discourse on integration in nations like France where the onus of becoming and being 'French' is put on the shoulders of 'those who come in'. Interestingly, similar sentiments regarding the nation state and loyalty to it echo within the geographical space of the Indian nation. Inadvertent comments by locals, nurses feel, are indications of their attitudes towards the migrants. Diana's claim that she has equal rights over the capital city of Delhi just as anybody else (quoted earlier) is part of a defence to such attitudes perceived by her as threatening. During interviews, discussions on their lives in Delhi revealed that opinions like that of Monica, a Punjabi woman in my neighbourhood, are heard often enough, and these lead to feelings of solidarity towards ethnic identities. Although Monica's statement—'...you South Indians are loyal to your state even when you are staying in Delhi...'—can be discounted as the opinion of just one person, this can have a strong impact on those who hear it, reminding one of the allegations by rightist discourses on Muslims in India. On the other hand, groups and associations formed by Malayalis can reach the level of 'parochialism'. But these can also be viewed in light of the resistance and response to the alienation they encounter in Delhi.

Malayali Associations

Malayali associations are registered associations under the Societies Registration Act and are often cultural associations that arrange get-togethers of people from Kerala. Here Kerala is that 'greater' Kerala which includes everyone who has an ancestral link to Kerala or whose parents spoke Malayalam or resided in Kerala before. People with mother tongues of Tamil, Tulu, Konkani or Malayalam can be members though what is required is an ultimate association with Kerala as a geographical and cultural space.

Office bearers of the Dwarka Malayalee Association, for example, describe the association as a collective interest group. This is the case with the Vikaspuri Malayali Association or Rohini Malayali Association. Office bearers, thus, prefer to register as a proactive group for Malayalis rather than for the entire locality. Identity politics is understated, though, in the association's practical relevance. Malayali associations in Delhi[13] are organised according to the concentration of Malayalis in various localities and the largest is the Delhi Malayali Association. All traditional hierarchies based on caste, religion, class and family status (*tarawad mahima*) continue to thrive within the group.

These associations are the bridges between Kerala and the host culture. They serve the important function of socialisation, familiarising oneself with fellow community members and cultural peculiarities. These associations run Malayalam classes for children and conduct training classes for music and dance forms popular in Kerala. Annual competitions on various forms of dance, music, oration, drawing, and painting, as also writing skills, are conducted by these organisations. Pankajam, a school teacher who lives in the neighbourhood of a colony where nurses of a private hospital stay (in Rohini Sector–3), says that her children are active in the cultural scene of the associations but keeps the relation at that level in order to avoid any kind of complication.

> ...Our children look forward to the annual competition organised by various organisations like Jansanskriti... We do not go for any other function due to lack of time for participation but our children prepare and go for the competitions...We also encourage it as this is the forum where they interact with other Malayali children and learn the language as well. We keep away from intense interaction with the community members...

However, some nurses in the study, Mariamma and Susanna, for instance, say that their children have not been active in the association scene. They attribute this to their lack of interest and lack of time due to work. Young nurses too say that they are not active in the functioning of the associations though they do attend the functions organised by the associations.

It must be clarified that when one says that there is a Malayali association, it is an all-male association. One is reminded of the 'men who play' in George's (2000) study of the US, who talked about the strategies of men to regain the status they lost because they are mere nurses' husbands. As the joint secretary of the Dwarka Malayalee Association put it, the association does provide reputation to those who actively participate in its functioning. Men who are active at the association level are considered prominent in terms of caste and monetary status in the local community.

There is a separate women's wing in some associations. This is a very 'generous' gesture because women are not meant to be office bearers. They are incorporated because of the contribution they make towards cultural programmes during celebrations and festivals, and also in teaching dance and music (the main cultural activities). And, of course, how can a function like Onam be complete without a round of *Thiruvathira*[14] performed by the women? Apart from this, what are the other functions that women perform? They are part of the *thalappoli* (in a decorative role), which is to welcome dignitaries or the god, where women stand in line in customary dress as time-honoured symbols of salutation to welcome the guest. There is little more to the 'role of women' in Malayali associations in Delhi.[15]

Sumi, one respondent who works as a nurse in a Delhi government hospital, is very aware of the gendered nature of the associations but does not think that she has any role to play in changing it:

> ...[laughing]... They [men] are interested in playing a leading role [in the community]...they do it all with such enthusiasm...and in any case where do women have time once they are married?... Being unmarried, we are not supposed to be there with those men either...

Festivals

As mentioned earlier, organising festivals like Onam and other celebrations like Ayyappa Pooja, Christmas and Easter are the main contributions of the Malayali association. Onam is celebrated generally on the first Sunday after the actual date has passed. However, the date is decided according to the convenience of the local Malayali population. Information about planning meetings is spread by word of mouth and through notices. Though meetings are open to all Malayalis, they are often attended only by the office bearers, who decide the date and venue by looking at the calendar of public holidays, school examinations and other such events to ensure maximum participation.

The venue is often a community hall or a public park determined by accessibility. As Reena's brother says:

> ...Onam, Christmas... these are the main festivals for us here [here indicates sector 3, Rohini, in this case] ... We organise a feast in the traditional way for Onam... There is a Malayali Association... but it is not very active except for organising festivals and is loosely structured... as all the members (men) work in offices or shops...no one has the time to work for it...'

What is the nature of the space? It is not exactly a public space that is open and accessible to all citizens, regardless of gender, race, ethnicity, age or socio-economic level. It is restricted in its access, and excludes others based on linguistic and ethnic characteristics. Yet, this already contextualised social space may appear neutral to those who are present. In fact, it even appears friendly to them because, unlike a public space as in public transport or on the streets, one's motives are not strictly personal; rather, one is powered by the fact that one is wanted and invited as part of a community and are gathered there for a special purpose.[16]

Nevertheless, festivals and celebrations of this nature are the only time the community gathers. The participation of women in this space has derived its meaning from rituals and practices over decades and even centuries. The emphasis on family in these collective events is probably why these events are designed as a space for families rather than individuals. That also probably adds to the discomfort of single women, like nurses. Single men, too, do not seem to occupy a full status unlike older men whose status as husband and father provides them with a rightful place in the community along with the status that age brings.

Just like the associations, the festival venue is a male space. At least, it is understood as a male space by some participants like Sumi:

> ...[laughing]... we [women] do not organise...and they [men] do all the organising business. It is their work... We pay for the feast[17]

> ...go for the function, take part in the feast and come back.... Sometimes we do not even go for the meetings to organise the get-together... What will we (women) do there? ...where there are so many men.

She says, supported by three other nurses, that they do not perceive themselves as part of the main/male space due to consciousness of norms of gender seclusion in the public space even while exercising more economic freedom and choice as workers in Delhi. This, by their own admission, saves them from labouring in community events which they describe as 'thankless' work. Unlike the men, the women nurses in my study do not find it useful to organise community events. This is understandable because they use the space as gendered beings who attribute it with meanings.[18] In a patriarchal society like that of India, women (like the other genders) infer different meanings about space, its use and the meaning it has for them. This hesitant attitude may be what is reflected in the segregated physical space occupied by women and men during festival celebrations.

Their ambivalent relationship with the community space does not diminish the hope that is placed on the 'omnipresence' of this community. Nevertheless, a differentiation between this faceless community and their individual contacts—friends, neighbours in Kerala and colleagues—pilots their approach in dealing with the identity politics within the community.

Weekly markets in the locality are another place to meet and exchange news. Markets function for a few hours from around 5 pm till 10 pm. This interaction is not very regular since they may visit the markets at different times every week. This is the time to discuss politics and the weather in Kerala, inform them about the dance class that was started by a Malayali teacher in the next neighbourhood and invite someone to drop in next Sunday.

Another regular place where interaction takes place is the 'south Indian shop' which functions as an ethnic market. Among themselves, south Indians refer to these shops as Malayali or Kerala shops or Tamil shops, depending on the shopkeeper's home state. These shops sell all the ingredients required for the culturally-specific food they are used to and that are important in maintaining their Malayali-ness.

Their interaction with migrant Malayalis other than nurses in Delhi happens on Sundays in church and during other religious occasions in churches and temples like St Thomas Church or the Ayyappa temple in R.K. Puram, the Sacred Heart Cathedral at Gole dak khana, the Uttara Guruvayur temple in Mayur Vihar in east Delhi, or the Ayyappa temple in Rohini in west Delhi.

The literature on migrant communities discusses the processes by which the migrants recreate the cultural contexts of their original settings. Print and electronic media facilitate this in more than one way. Thus, Asianet has become the common name for the Malayalam channels though there are more than eight of them. Malayalam newspapers—*Malayala Manorama* and *Mathrubhoomi*—started Delhi editions of their Malayalam news dailies to cater to the Malayali readership here. These have started informing the Malayali identity and defining it by keeping the community abreast of developments at 'home'.[19]

Two and Two Add up to Four? Individual Agency and Collective Action

The individual Malayali nurse's agency is evident in no small measure in her initiatives in getting trained as a nurse and the processes of migration to Delhi and the life there. Malayali and female networks help them in their choice of profession and the means to realise it, which is a form of agency that is collective. They also look for relative professional autonomy (though not all of them express it openly), which is less articulated and therefore undeveloped. They bridge the gap between seemingly disconnected issues of their ethnic and linguistic identities within the larger legalities of universal citizenship. However, there has been no collective action among nurses based on their linguistic or ethnic identities, though many such plans emerged among them at various points.[20] Considering the many obstacles they face in terms of housing and other practical needs, they have not mobilised despite the long tradition of nurses' migration from Kerala to Delhi. Nevertheless, their responses to challenges at the professional level are based on individual solutions. This issue came up in several discussions.

> ...There are many issues...Nurses migrate to Delhi or any other place from Kerala under severe constraints... We have to tackle our lives here and work in shifts that are not easy... When we come to Delhi we also learn [simultaneously] to deal with language, a different city, work culture and we also have to look for better opportunities...Life is not secure enough for us to indulge in fights...

Clara who has been with AIIMS does have a more secure professional life than the nurses in the private sector. But her words do reflect the almost universal opinion of nurses in the study that their priority here is not to improve the conditions of their existence in Delhi; such an attitude being shaped by larger realities around their lives and work here. Clara is representative of the other nurses in the study who also look at migration as an inevitable part of their life, not always stemming out after collective action but as something that is seen as a solution to their search for better lives.

The conditions of their existence in Delhi also invite comparisons with Kerala hospitals—the majority believe that nurses' service conditions and status are really poor in Kerala. Political activism for professional purposes is almost absent in Kerala, as pointed out by Molly O.S., president of the Kerala Government Nurses' Association.[21] George has explored the effective absence of political mobilisation of nurses in Kerala as well (2005: 54). And this also pulls them back from any kind of collective action and a sense of fatalism that seems to be in their minds. Moreover, differences in training, competition to get to the best position despite the network, lack of belief in the capacity of the state to improve their working lives and the trusted path of migration abroad are cited as reasons for not insisting on mobilisation.

Recently, there have been attempts to mobilise Malayali nurses in the form of the Malayali Nurses Welfare Association (MNWA) by a non-nurse, Usha Krishnakumar, who has been actively associated with the Indian National Congress. However, it is the strikes mainly by migrant nurses in the private nursing homes and hospitals in Delhi during December 2009–January 2010 that attracted the attention of the media and the Delhi government to some extent (Nair 2010: 23–25). These strikes also brought to light the increasing gap in service conditions between private and public sector hospitals in Delhi. Most importantly, these strikes highlighted for the first time certain issues that are specifically relevant for migrant nurses like curtailment of mobility and freedom to take leave, within the rule, to go out of Delhi and so on. And these strikes also answered the critics on their point about nurses on complicity for their conditions. The question 'why do nurses not organise in the private sector despite the exploitative conditions of work?' has always been raised. These strikes showed that extraordinary determination is required for nurses to carry on any out-of-work protests due to lack of financial resources and the strategically played out pressure tactics of the hospital management. This becomes especially difficult in a city where they have limited networks.

Recent controversies that erupted when Indraprastha Apollo hospital took action against nurses who spoke in Malayalam during duty hours show that ethnic and linguistic peculiarities have to be hidden from the formal realm of the profession.[22] They illustrate that the modern universal citizen lives through her gender and ethnic identities every day. They do not necessarily make clear the connections between them, though they, as women workers, provide an example of negotiating the realm of Indian citizenship. They perceive a 'gaze' that is stern, hostile and disapproving—from the local population in Delhi, from non-nurses among the migrant Malayalis and from non-Malayali nurses. They try to make sense of the stigmatising experience through the binaries of 'we' and 'they'. The primary collective identity is explained through these binaries—nurses and others, Malayalis and Hindi speakers, men and 'us'. Of these the first and the last are largely played out within the identity politics of the migrant community.

Issues of language, which also measure their professional competence, are put to the test by patients and the hospital staff. The nurses in my study also feel that there has been a growing tendency in Delhi hospitals to reject the candidature of Malayali nurses through informal means, by casual remarks like 'anyway you people will leave soon'. Malayali nurses' Hindi accents and their supposed lack of fluency in English and Hindi are quoted as reasons not to employ them. While problems with both spoken Hindi and English are to some extent true, they are also praised for being able to pick up other languages quickly. Malayali nurses complain that despite the problems of language and accent that Manipuri nurses have in Delhi, they are increasingly preferred over Malayali nurses in many hospitals in the city.

The medical superintendent in a Delhi government hospital told me on conditions of anonymity when I went for permission to interview nurses inside the hospitals:[23]

> ... I can guarantee that Kerala nurses are the best nurses. They are obedient, they are nice and create no problem. I am a North Indian but I have seen that nurses from this place (north India) do not work but they "sweet talk" you into believing that they do everything...Malayali nurses work really hard, are very sympathetic to patients... I have seen patients asking specially for Kerala nurses.

Some nurses in the sample think they work harder and believe that favouritism towards nurses from the north does exist.

Patients too are reported to be less demanding with nurses from the north. Ethnicity and language, along with class, are thus experienced as markers of overt discrimination.

Malayali nurses' incessant quest for greener pastures has been noticed by hospitals in Delhi. It affects the quality of patient care, as experienced nurses fly off to distant lands, forcing the hospitals to invest in training a new batch. This is said to be the reason why Malayali nurses fall out of grace with administrators and managers in Delhi hospitals and nursing schools. Some nurses in my sample have also complained that nurses from other parts of India are now seriously challenging their earlier 'monopoly' in the Delhi hospitals. Nurses from Manipur and the Hindi-speaking northern states are now being favoured.

However hard Malayali nurses defend themselves in terms of the quality of their work, there is no questioning of the fact that in the past few years the transnational migration of nurses has increased momentously. Delhi hospitals are, therefore, under pressure to retain their trained nurses.[24] Salaries and service conditions have improved, though only marginally. Hospitals are also taking other measures like paying overtime and offering hostels for single women. They have initiated the system of entering into a bond or contract with the nurses to ensure service periods of two to three years; should they leave before that, nurses have to forgo the security deposit and provident fund that are with the hospitals.

As a researcher alert to all forms of constraints and control on workers, I looked to nurses' responses to such contracts. Surprisingly, the nurses whom I interviewed paid little interest to their contracts with the hospitals;[25] rather they turned it to their advantage in their plans for the next phase of migration. They calculate their period of stay in terms of the time required to prepare for their tests to go abroad and to earn the mandatory years of experience for work in a foreign hospital. Mridula is clear about her priorities. She says:

> ...It does not really matter. I need to stay in Delhi for at least two years because if I apply to the Ministry of Health hospitals in Saudi Arabia or Kuwait, I need to show that I have worked for at least these many years in a technologically advanced hospital... I am also planning to prepare for the IELTS examinations...This or that plan should work in my favour...My first preference is the US, then Ireland or other parts in Europe, and in case I don't make

it, I will look for opportunities in the Gulf...I am ready to go to
the Gulf only if they are the government hospitals...I will take the
interviews and written examinations for them...A batch just left
now, last week for Kuwait...I will not work here forever...

Smitha, who was with a charitable hospital in north-west Delhi,
and who got through the test and interview for the post of
staff nurse in a Kuwait government-sponsored contract left the
night of her last day of duty. She neither informed the hospital
nor did she bother to collect her money from the hospital, which
would have required a formal resignation in advance. She was
bound to work for two years in the hospital in Punjabi Bagh and
had just completed a year, having worked for two years in another
hospital in east Delhi. The systematic way in which she went
about preparing for her trip to Kuwait is subversive, because the
hospital did not have a clue about her and three of her friends
who were flying out of Delhi after completing their night duty.
She had been shopping for the past three months and her luggage
was packed a week before she left. Extra clothes and other things
were sent back to her family through a nurse who was visiting
Kerala; other things were given to friends. For a woman who had
been sheltered from the outside world by parents and for someone who was taking her first flight, she betrayed no anxiety.
Instead, she was full of enthusiasm that her plans about coming
to Delhi were now half-fulfilled.

Smitha was completely defiant about the agreement that
she had signed when she joined the hospital and told me how
irrelevant the hospital contract looked to her now:

> I do not care about the money. What is left with them (management)
> is less than one month's salary in Kuwait. They pay us so little
> and expect us to be loyal? They treat us as if we have no other
> place to go. It (the contract she signed) has no importance as far
> as I am concerned. Now I just want to reach the new hospital
> and join duty as soon as possible. I am leaving this evening with
> three others from here and we will join duty next week... I will
> tell my friends that they should come soon too.

Her attitude is typical of those who were leaving, like Sindhu
who was going to Ireland. At that point at least, the Malayali
diaspora and its patriarchal attitudes were of no significance to
their immediate lives. They focused single-mindedly on their

plans where only family, friends and global visa policies mattered. This life strategy is focused, rebellious of the established class norms and based on hard and 'smart' work.[26] Young women use their earnings for progress in their professional lives,[27] thus postponing their decision to save for their marriages. Yet, many facets of their lives synchronise faith in the rationality of the individual on one hand and reluctance in coming together to face the challenges and injustices as nurses, as single women and as migrants on the other.

There is, therefore, a definite absence of collective will on the part of Malayali nurses, despite attempts at mobilisation. As migrant single women workers, their concerns are numerous. Returning to the patriarchal context of nurses in the original home and Delhi as an extension of that, forming an 'authentic' part of the 'greater' Kerala, dowry is a price women pay to have been born as women. Anti-dowry movements and legislations changed the context only to the extent that dowry is now called 'gifts' and women think that they deserve their parents' share of the property when they leave their natal homes. Nurses are known for saving their salaries 'at the cost of their health and well being' for dowry. As we have discussed, they defer the decision to marry in favour of a migratory opportunity abroad. Dowry still remains intact in the wider schema and there have not been any collective pronouncements or plans of action by the nurses to fight the evil. Correspondingly, as migrant women they face a number of challenges in Delhi, including finding accommodation and the mindset of the local and migrant population alike.

It is not inappropriate to mention an incident that illustrates the assumptions regarding a single woman nurse who travels alone and the extent of her vulnerability. Dhanya, a nurse working with a mission hospital in south-east Delhi, was going on vacation to Kerala. On the journey, some male Malayali passengers started talking to her; they asked her name, where she worked and family details which, in the Indian context, are common exchanges. When she came back to work, she started getting phone calls at the hostel asking whether she remembered the person on the train and whether she would like to go out with him. When she refused, a group of men waited outside the hostel gate on Sundays when she was going to church with her friends. When the men threatened the girls, the hostel had to call the police. The matter did not end there; fellow nurses began spreading stories that she must actually have been an 'adventurous' woman during her trip.

We have seen several examples of networks of friends and colleagues, almost exclusively Malayalis, who are part of their everyday lives and are the stand-in family in critical times. But these networks are a contingent collection of individuals. Collective action involves acting together to improve service conditions and fight institutionalised discrimination in its various forms. This has not emerged, and needs to be probed further given the eminent role that collective action has played in their home state of Kerala in improving state policies, as Kurien (1995) points out.

Malayali Women, Delhi and the (Re)emergence of 'Kerala Model' of Patriarchy

Larger frameworks and dominant gender practices that support Malayali cultural spaces in Delhi provide the understanding of a highly patriarchal context for nurses' lives therein. That kind of discourse is not understood nor seen as important. This remains more or less the same as that of the *pedakozhi koovunna kalam* (when the hen begins to crow). Any suggestion that a woman has the right to public space is met with resistance as in the fascinating study by Tamale (1999) titled *When Hens Begin to Crow* on gender and politics in Uganda. In many African cultures, a crowing hen is considered an omen of bad news of adverse times ahead and a woman candidate for the 1996 general election was shouted at: 'Do hens crow?' In Kerala one of the signs of *kaliyugam*[28] is the superciliousness that the women are assumed to demonstrate when they have power, which is a sign that bad times are approaching. The message here is that women have no business in the public space, outside the domestic sphere. It is in this context that questions of the identity politics of nurses revolve around questions of gender.

Many nurses, however, make space for themselves in their new situation in Delhi and express their dissatisfaction with the way their family, especially male members, try to exercise control. These are subtle subversions that can make patriarchy adjust its frame a little. These appear as expressions of frustration over their physical and social movements in Kerala and may not, at that stage, be references to men's patriarchal power over their sexuality and body. Yet, they recognise the concern with respectability and the ease with which women acquire 'a bad name' should she venture out alone and get implicated. Shijy says:

> My Papa is so strict that I feel like saying that I would have stayed in Kerala had he not been there. He never used to allow me even to meet my friends... and just to visit the neighbour he would ask my mother to accompany me...

Suja makes it clear that reputation is not just the concern of parents but that, as young women, they have something at stake too.

> In Kerala I was not allowed to go anywhere (outside the home) without someone—brother or father or at least mother. But here I go alone to the market, to buy vegetables, other food items and clothes. I also go with my friends to meet other friends working in other hospitals. I come alone at 8 or even 9 o'clock at night. Nothing happens to me... But if I did that in Kerala it would be a scandal. Neighbours would talk about my character...it does not matter whether I am good or bad... I prefer to stay here than staying at home...

This chaperoning, if not policing, of young nurses carried out by parents in Kerala is taken over by the Malayali community in Delhi. Therefore, opinions like those of Mohanan Pillai (quoted earlier) are 'disseminated' with a certain sense of legitimacy. Interestingly, the role of women's networks in this area also brings up some attention-grabbing scenarios. From a new hairstyle to new friendships, every change and movement is under scrutiny by the networks that often act as chaperones. I was also able to observe a few episodes of feuds and cold wars between the women, which had to do with the subject of control by the 'more powerful' within the group and resistance to it. These observations helped me contextualise these networks as originating and reproducing themselves in the cultural and patriarchal contexts of the Malayali community. They help in the negotiation between at least three different spaces at different times in Delhi: the professional space, interactions with the migrant community and local places.

While most of them project their vulnerability to any possibility of disrepute to their family, there exists a sense of balance between the emotion and economy in their relations with the family. Most of them feel that earning power gives more power to their words: '...that is natural. When one is economically independent, people listen to her/his words (carefully)' says Annamma Vijayan (47 years old at the time of interview).

Nurses experience greater freedom and independence in Delhi, which is a source of achievement and a result of their hard work. Their status as workers brings new confidence as they move around in Delhi, looking for better service conditions and salaries in hospitals all over, and possibly beyond.

Women nurses in my sample have fairly strong perceptions of identity, both as women and as migrants, within the spaces of the professional institutions and migrant communities. As in all groups, their identities are shaped in response to that of the other, who is dominant and male. Delhi is a transit residence suspended between 'home' and elsewhere. This brings ambivalence to their responses to their own identity formation in opposition to the obstacles they face. This aspect of their existence leads to a peculiar relation to time—though many of them stay for a long time, they perceive Delhi as never really theirs. We saw this ambivalence in their relationship with the community. The Malayali community and its leadership are defined by male worldviews. Their negotiations with this take the form of using the exclusive quality of their very marginality within the migrant community to pursue their goals, both professional and personal, which are bargains with patriarchy.

Nurses provide interesting insights into the agency-structure debate, realising significant changes in their situation while reinforcing accepted norms, especially gender relations. What is interesting about the migrant Malayali context in Delhi is that their negotiation with the community also happens at the professional level, particularly with a lack of clarity on the status that they are ready to grant nurses. On the one hand, it is the favourite profession of not one but many; on the other, nurses are always reminded that they have to be apologetic to be what they are, namely, nurses. Thus, there seems to be an invisible pact between nurses and the community. Possibilities of inspection and deferred judgements and pre-trial warnings over the moral character loom large over the community of nurses, thus signalling the (re)establishment of the 'Kerala model' of patriarchy in Delhi. This community chaperoning is the amulet or the talisman that Malayalis, especially women, have to wear for protection wherever they are.

This chapter has tried to show the complexities of relocation within the Indian territory, where legal issues of settling down are clearly laid out and relocation can be taken for granted due to citizenship rights. Despite those assumptions of universal, unmarked citizenship as envisioned in the liberal framework of the Indian constitution, ethnic and gender identities emerge as major issues for my respondents at all major junctures of decision making. These identities act as facilitators as well as constraints in their relationship with the new city and its residents, fellow migrants and colleagues. There is contradiction and ambivalence in claiming the public space, which is seen as belonging to men, thus demonstrating the power of the public-domestic binary in the Malayali consciousness.

Notes

1. This chapter is imagined and construed as contributing towards the understanding of nurses' lives as a whole. It touches upon various issues that may appear peripheral but are seen to have a deep influence on nurses' lives and on the ways in which they plan their future in the current physical and social space. Various categories emerged in their narrations and prominent among them were the Malayalis themselves (discussed later). Not everyone was forthcoming on these issues from fear of appearing opinionated and biased. And yet whatever the views expressed by the nurses are worth presenting to the readers in order to give them an idea of the lives of nurses. This chapter is defined not so much by the methodology but serves the purpose of contributing towards the presentation of the nurses' lives in Delhi.

2. Trans: When Mahabali was ruling (Kerala), people were equal. There were no lies, fraud, cheating or theft. The legend goes like this: The geographical area which constitutes the present Kerala or a part of it became a very prosperous and egalitarian 'kingdom' under the rule of the *asura*/evil king Mahabali. *Devas* (gods) became very jealous of his popularity and were afraid that he would take over their position as the invincible. So the devas plotted against Mahabali and, as usual, Indra, the lord of the devas, masterminded a plot to dethrone him. Vishnu, heeding the pleas of the devas, took his fifth avatar as Vamana and sent Mahabali to *pathala* (underground kingdom of the asuras) by crooked means unknown till then in the latter's kingdom of Kerala.

3. Probably it is also mixed—modern and pre-modern—imaginations coming together to form the base of a patrifocal notion that single women needing to migrate to earn a living does not fit with the imagined space of Kerala where 'all is well'.

4. Of both Malayali men and women. It is important here to point out that single men also are seen to be facing the issue of not having problems of 'adult status' in a family-oriented community space. More of this is discussed in the section about festivals later in this chapter.

5. She reported that she would have preferred a confrontational path against these men who are identified as a social nuisance by everyone but that her parents reminded her 'it would ultimately put her in trouble because "she was the one who had something (reputation) to lose".'

6. For an understanding of Malayalam cinema's stardom and its image in Malayali minds, see Osella and Osella (2006: 169–202).

7. The failure of the state to follow the federally-promoted Mahalanobis model of the second Five-Year Plan fame and advance the agenda of heavy industrialisation and therefore the very low level of employment opportunities in the secondary sector in Kerala have been highly criticised in Kerala. The progressiveness of the Malayali demographic profile in contrast to this led to debates by theoreticians across the world on the phenomenon that they thought as not common and was termed as an alternative model of development.

8. See the section 'Love, Sex and the Modern Family' for a historical understanding of the discourse in Kerala in Devika (2005: 356–61).

9. Utsavam and perunnal are festivals celebrated at the local level; some myths and stories associated with them make sense only to the village and others have relevance to the 'greater traditions' of Hinduism or Christianity and go beyond the cultural specificity of Kerala.

10. Bargain of giving into the norms of patriarchy and gaining respectability in society.

11. Mohanan Pillai's case is something I want to illustrate with the quote where he tries to show himself as someone seeking to claim the 'unofficial' gatekeeper role to the world of nurses that I was trying to enter.

12. While this example may appear simplistic, it shows solidarity with one's own ethnic group and this practice is not specific to Malayalis. (Re)appearances of ethnic and linguistic identities at a parochial level have been in the news in all regions of India, leading to riots and physical assault on minorities, the latest being in Maharashtra.

13. In fact, I was told that Malayali associations exist wherever Malayalis go and there is nothing peculiar about Delhi's case.

14. Thiruvathira is a traditional group dance, which is performed in the front yards of houses on Hindu festive occasions. Women, in even numbers, dance in circles to a theme-based song which they sing (nowadays, tape recorders are used instead). The song is often about a god or king.

15. As pointed out by some Malayali women, women are present in various functions of the Delhi Malayali Association.They teach dance, music and language. Of course, one does not disagree here. But why are there no women presidents or secretaries? There are cultural organisations of Malayalis like Jansanskriti that takes a progressive line on social issues, which has a woman president; but even there, it is more the exception than the rule.

16. Normally, discourses of women's right to public space proclaim it as rightfully belonging to women when they use it 'legitimately' and 'for a purpose'. This common understanding is found to be true by the study by Viswanath and Tandon-Mehrotra (2007: 1546) in the urban context of Delhi.

17. Food for the festivals and community events are prepared by men. Traditionally, male Brahmins were called in to cook vegetarian food for Hindu homes and temples.

18. Studies have pointed out that the status of men, for example, is closely tied to different life rituals like marriage and fatherhood and life chances like education, employment and ownership of property. Caroline Osella and Filippo Osella (2006: 208) state thus in the context of men and masculinity in Kerala: 'Men and women alike may find themselves circumscribed and required to make demanding performances of gender and heteronormativity.'

19. In fact, the news item in *Mathrubhoomi* are said to be 'all from Kerala', making it mandatory to subscribe to an English newspaper in order to know what is happening in Delhi.

20. One reason why this question comes up in many discussions has to do with well-known, successful trade union traditions in Kerala and the history of localised collective action among communities and interest groups in Kerala.

21. Molly says that breaking out of this 'apolitical' nature of mobilisation is one of her objectives in Kerala. From the discussions on her paper 'Nurses as Women Workers in the Public Sector Hospitals', presented in the national seminar on Indian Nursing in the New Era of Healthcare, 2-3 December 2010, New Delhi.

22. In fact, this issue was touched upon by nurses in the recent strikes. This issue received coverage in national dailies too. See, for example, 'Caught speaking Malayalam, Apollo nurses asked to resign', ExpressIndia.com, 26 May 2009.

23. As I wrote in the section on the field and my methods of research, I tried to access nurses from many angles, using snowball techniques.

I went through doctors, accessing them in the departments and wards they controlled and then going through the connections made available to me by the nurses. Sometimes, when I went through formal channels, I was denied permission.

24. One must, however, add that the hospitals have always benefited from the flow of fresh GNM holders. This stream of nurses has been continuous from Kerala and has acted as a permanent and reliable stock in times of shortages and helped the management cut costs as these nurses were paid low wages in the name of their lack of experience.

25. Most male nurses whom I have spoken,brought this up as an issue. However, nurses till now have been subversive in their dealings with the contract.

26. Reminding one of the 'self-help' books and inspirational preachers, Anusha who always advocates the importance of the nurse's own role in improving her status, says: 'You have to do smart work and not just hard work'.

27. This is a significant difference between the older generation and the younger ones in my sample. I refrain from extending it to nurses in general because many older nurses migrated to the US, the UK and other countries through their own efforts from the 1960s onwards; so what the younger nurses in my study are doing is not extraordinary. However, I am trying to argue that the younger nurses in my sample, in comparison to the older ones, defer saving for dowry and instead save to invest in better job opportunities, and defer the decision to find security in marriage to a later stage. Apart from rescheduling saving for the purpose of dowry, many pointed out that they needed the money for their preparations to go abroad and thus deferred their 'saving for the family' role as well.

28. 'Age of Kali' (demon kali and not the goddess kali), 'age of vice' is one of the four stages of development that the world goes through as part of the cycle of Yugas, as described in the Brahminical scriptures, the others being *Satya Yuga, Treta Yuga* and *Dwapara Yuga.* All religions that originated in India like Hinduism, Buddhism and Sikhism recognise this time frame that is traditionally thought to last 432,000 years. According to this belief, human civilisation degenerates spiritually throughout the *Kaliyugam* and so this age is referred to as the Dark Age.

Conclusion

Along with Filipinos and Sri Lankans, Indian nurses form one of the largest groups of migrant women workers in the international service sector. Such migration has led to a situation where First World women's labour is being replaced by that of Third World women. The shortage of workers in industrialised countries is a result of reduced interest of the local population towards nursing as a profession, for reasons that include the spread of non-curable diseases like HIV/AIDS.[1] Nursing is thus part of a restructured international division of labour with its hierarchies and forms of exploitation. This study seeks to locate the agency and life strategies of women from Kerala shaped by these evolving labour markets, linking the global South and North, as discussed in Khadria (2006), considerations of status of profession and service conditions in their home country.

Malayali nurses form the largest chunk of nurses who migrate from India, looking for job opportunities abroad. Better salaries and terms and conditions of work are the attraction. As we have seen, nurses cite unemployment within Kerala, low salaries and poor working conditions in the hospitals and nursing homes in India, as also the negative work environment as primary contributing factors that push them to leave. Some also mention a desire to travel and see the world, or learn a new language, apart from the ability to earn a living and become self-reliant as the motivation. Ever since modern nursing was institutionalised in India, Malayali nurses have been its main recruits, given their early access to modern education and the compulsions to earn a regular income. Kerala has a very vibrant nursing education sector, both public and private, that was recognised by the Kerala Nurses and Midwives Council. But the immediate availability of jobs and increasing migration opportunities have augmented the demand for nursing courses, beyond what this state can provide.

As a result, apart from getting trained in Kerala, Malayali women travel to join nursing schools in Tamil Nadu, Andhra Pradesh,

Karnataka and Delhi. Some also receive training in newer schools in Maharashtra, Uttar Pradesh and Punjab. This study has, therefore, highlighted how for many Malayali women the life strategy to become a nurse implies a decision to migrate for education. But precisely because the choice to study nursing is part of a larger set of strategies, many women create 'blueprints' of their future professional and personal lives, replete with plans for each stage. Their years in Delhi constitute only one of the stages along the journey that is envisioned.

As the chapters charting the history of nursing have shown, the first nursing recruits came from backgrounds of destitution and poverty. This image of nurses as needy and poor has persisted despite positive developments in the general economic situation of Kerala and changes in the class background of nursing candidates. What is particularly denigrating to the status of the profession is the poor general working conditions of nurses in Indian hospitals and nursing homes. With the exception of the public sector, salaries are much below the prescribed minimum wages, with no match between their post-secondary level of education and working status.

Status anxiety has thus been the most important problem in Indian nursing, where low economic remuneration combines perniciously with social prejudice. Notions of purity and pollution in the Indian context, so entangled with the caste system, stigmatises anyone dealing with bodily fluids. In the case of nurses, who handle sick bodies, the stigma is heightened. The gendered nature of their work as providers of care further diminishes its value. So-called feminine attributes of compassion and kindness get prioritised, which are then delinked from their work. The fact that they have to work with strangers, including men, and that too at night, raises questions about their character, thus turning a nurse bride into the last choice for grooms from 'good' families. Culturally 'inappropriate' uniforms in overcrowded hospitals are perceived to have caused tremendous pressures on these women, who often share the conservative cultural values of their patients and the general public.

Despite the specificities of the Indian cultural context, it is worth remembering that the stigmatisation of nursing is global. One solution in India has been to displace its worst aspects by appointing helpers and ayahs. More generally, the increasing use of technological equipment in medical treatment has helped nursing professionalise itself to some degree, though this route is only available in a few of Delhi's hospitals. Whatever changes have taken place in Delhi's health sector through the entry of global capital and corporate-style hospitals, these changes have not translated into improved working conditions for nurses. Rather, hospital managements routinely cut costs by keeping the wages of nurses and other lower-level employees to a minimum. Other sources of discontentment include control mechanisms to restrict the professional mobility of nurses which include confiscating nursing certificates at the time of their joining a hospital, and signing of 'bonds' with unfavourable contractual terms and conditions. One has only to compare this situation with those of consultant physicians, whose exorbitant salaries and free movement remind nurses on a daily basis of the gulf between them.

While I was writing this book, Delhi witnessed a series of nurses' strikes in 2009 and early 2010. These strikes spread across various private hospitals, and seem to have been triggered by the implementation of revised pay scales following the Government of India's Sixth Pay Commission recommendation in public sector hospitals, which made the already extensive disparities in the salaries of nurses even more glaring. Apart from the fact that the labour laws in public sector institutions minimise the exploitation of their workforce, nurses have at different points made efforts at collective bargaining where Malayali nurses, admittedly, cannot be attributed much participation. The issues that have received publicity were severe cases of sexual assault and harassment, the demand for a change of uniform, and so on. Yet, as this study has shown, leaders in the profession have been consistently concerned to improve the status of nursing by finding a better place within the Indian health sector. The nurses' professional association—the Trained Nurses Association of India—began by forwarding petitions on a range of issues, before the public sector nurses formed a union of their own. The struggle of nurses in India has also been one of overcoming its colonial legacy and finding an 'Indian' identity, as we saw in the campaign over uniforms.

Nurses are also fighting for their sense of personhood within their social circles and everyday worlds. One can see that the drive to improve status, image and service conditions brings in a feminist dimension. Beyond the obvious fact that this is a profession dominated by women, it is the constraints set by collective prejudice, social and professional norms on their public lives that require feminist analyses.

Social prejudices—often operating through rumour and gossip—are said to be at the foundation of a nurse's distress. Kerala, as it is being reproduced among its migrants in Delhi, has not lost its characteristics as a rural, patriarchal community. The anxiety that is felt when the existing gender and class hegemony is challenged by the presence of nurses—who are seen as 'unrestrained' sexual beings—is resolved by stigmatising and stereotyping the group which, consciously or unconsciously, challenges these hegemonies. While many of them present the freedom they enjoy in Delhi in tangible terms, they are clearly constrained by their need to bargain with the patriarchal system, both within the migrant community and with the local population. Eager to prove that they are dutiful daughters and sisters who do not malign the family name and honour, their discourses on independence, career and freedom are groomed to fit into the highly patriarchal Malayali nuclear family that is the norm in Kerala.

Nurses respond to these challenges by forming and finding refuge in their own networks. These networks are constituted by peer groups, and women from similar socio-economic and working backgrounds, who are the main source of information on nursing education, job opportunities and migration processes within India and abroad. As we have seen, such networks are crucial for getting jobs, moving to Delhi, finding residential quarters, and coping with the stress of starting life in a strange city. They figure prominently in further migration plans. While networks betray an ambivalent attitude towards migrant community politics, they respond, however, most often by conforming to the wider social norms, thus exerting peer pressure on young nurses to follow the accepted practices within the group.

This study highlights the dynamics of the lives of migrant Malayali nurses in Delhi, which, in turn, is linked to their plans to migrate further. With more information available on conditions elsewhere, nurses plan keeping all possibilities in mind. This is done at the time these women are studying nursing. Nurses today are quite aware of the fluctuating nature of international visa opportunities and the opening up of labour markets in various parts of the world. Many of them look at their exposure to technological facilities in Delhi's bigger hospitals as training experience that is compulsory for applying abroad. Coaching institutes for English tests that have sprung up in Delhi in recent years target nurses as a major group. Young nurses in this study invest in these training courses, postponing their financial investments in marriage—experienced as a compulsory institution in their lives—to a later stage.

Questions of status that have been frequently discussed throughout this study raise further issues of relevance for state policy. To begin with, there is the heterogeneous and chaotic nature of institutions of health care in Delhi, which are largely unregulated. State policy is also ambiguous on the question of migration though shortage of nurses has and remains a major concern for the state. The hierarchy within nursing—BSc Nursing, GNM and ANM—is a consequence of its professionalisation, but has made collective bargaining difficult. In order to tackle the exploitation of all those who work in the health sector as nursing workers it is necessary to recognise the under-qualified workforce that makes up its unorganised segments. Thus, instead of demanding their elimination, under-qualified nurses need to find inclusion within regularisation drives for the better enforcement of rules, working conditions and salaries. This would go a long way towards mitigating shortages of nursing staff for nursing services in Indian hospitals.

Nurses said frequently: 'Who would go to a foreign country, leaving their home, with enough work and decent working conditions?' This reflects the interconnections between nurses' migration, their identity as belonging to India, their status within the country, the state of global markets for health workers and the wider national and international policies on workers' movement.

This study has sought to break the silence that surrounds Malayali nurses' lives as migrant women. A holistic understanding includes both the personal and professional dimensions of their lives, especially in terms of the challenges posed to single women migrants. Such an approach, focussing on different aspects of their lived experiences, in fact reveals how the identities of gender, class and ethnicity unmask the claims of national citizenship which is the topic for an altogether separate discussion. Delhi is also the site where the Malayali diaspora enables patriarchy to play an important mediating role among its members. Kerala's cultural context is recreated in Delhi and traditional patterns of interaction are followed here too, sometimes reinforcing gender relations. A Malayali nurse's life strategy in Delhi is, therefore, shaped at the intersections offered by processes and plans of migration, negotiating everyday life in the community and the status offered by her work in contemporary society.

Note

1. Personal communication with Anne Verne, a nurse turned health consultant in Paris, France. (Name changed on request.)

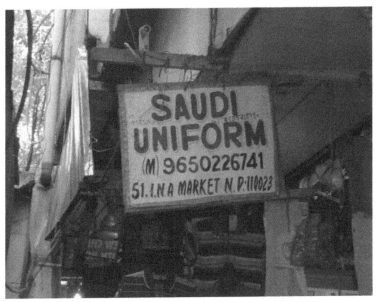

Note: Delhi facilitates Malayali nurses' migration abroad by offering information and opportunities. This tailoring shop, one of the many in INA Market in South Delhi—a popular market for Malayali nurses—is symbolic of the ways in which Delhi assists nurses in preparation for their lives ahead abroad.

Source: Photograph by the author.

Appendix

Information on Nurses Who were Part of the Study

S. No.	Name*	Age	Workplace/Names of hospitals**	Educational qualification***	Marital status/Accommodation	Religion/Caste****
1	Diana Johnson	31	SGR/pvt	GNM	Married/rented	Chr/RC
2	Bindu P.K.	26	SGR/pvt	GNM	Unmarried/rented	Hindu/Nair
3	Beena Jacob	22	SGR/pvt	GNM	Unmarried/rented	Christian/RC
4	Mridula Mariam Thomas	24	SGR/pvt	GNM	Unmarried/hostel	Christian/Orth
5	Anusha Sarah Paulos	23	SGR/pvt	GNM	Unmarried/hostel	Christian/Orth
6	Marie Shaji	29	SGR/pvt	GNM	Married/hostel	Christian/RC
7	Sheeba Varkey	29	SGR/pvt	GNM	Married/own house	Christian/RC
8	Jancey James	28	SGR/pvt	GNM	Married	Christian/RC
9	Annie Chacko	31	SGR/pvt	GNM	Married	Christian/Pent
10	Sheila	39	SGR/pvt Gulf returned	GNM	Married/own house/husband in Kerala	Hindu/Nair
11	Bincy Joseph	23	SGR/pvt	B.Sc.	Unmarried/hostel	Christian/Orth

	Name	Age				Religion
12	Jessy Job	28	SGR/pvt	GNM	Married/rented	Christian/RC
13	Lisy Varkey	26	SGR/pvt	GNM	Unmarried/ hostel	Christian/Orth
14	Betty Joseph	22	SGR/pvt	GNM	Unmarried/ hostel	Christian/RC
15	Julie Jacob	22	SGR/pvt	GNM	Unmarried/ hostel	Christian/RC
16	Sunita Narayanan	24	SGR/pvt	GNM	Unmarried/hostel	Hindu/Ezhava
17	Rajitha K. Sebastian	22	SM/pvt	GNM	Unmarried/hostel	Christian/RC
18	Meena Jacob	22	SM/pvt	GNM	Unmarried/hostel	Christian/Orth
19	Shalini	23	SM/pvt	GNM	Unmarried/hostel	Christian/RC
20	Binu	23	SM/pvt	GNM	Unmarried/hostel	Christian/RC
21	Reeja Philip	24	SM/pvt	GNM	Unmarried/hostel	Christian/RC
22	Rani Mathew	26	SM/pvt	GNM	Unmarried/hostel	Christian/RC
23	Divya Mathew	28	SM/pvt	GNM	Unmarried/hostel	Christian/RC
24	Shiny Joseph	22	SM/pvt	GNM	Unmarried/hostel	Christian/Orth
25	Bijitha Jacob	30	SM/pvt	GNM	Married/hostel, husband in KSEB Kerala/Child 4 years in Kerala	Christian/RC
26	Eliamma Kosi	26	SM/pvt	GNM	Unmarried	Christian/Orth
27	Mariamma	51	SM/pvt	GNM	Married/hostel/husband in Kerala (missionary)	Christian/Pent

(Continued)

Appendix (*Continued*)

S. No.	Name	Age	Workplace/Names of hospitals	Educational qualification	Marital status/Accommodation	Religion/Caste
28	Sally Joy	24	SM/pvt	GNM	Unmarried/hostel	Christian/RC
29	Myriam Baby	22	SM/pvt	GNM	Unmarried/hostel	Christian/RC
30	Bindumol P.R.	22	SM/pvt	GNM	Unmarried/hostel	Hindu/Ezhava
31	Rajimol Boban	23	SM/pvt	GNM	Unmarried/hostel	**Christian/Orth**
32	Rincy	24	JG/pvt	GNM	Unmarried/Hostel	**Christian/RC**
33	Babitha Jose	27	JG/pvt	GNM	Married/hostel/husband in Jhansi	Christian/Orth
34	Shijy George	23	JG/pvt	GNM	Unmarried/hostel	Christian/Pent
35	Sakshi George	25	JG/pvt	GNM	Unmarried/hostel	Christian/RC
36	Molamma Kurien	23	JG/pvt	GNM	Unmarried/hostel	Christian/RC
37	Jeena Jacob	26	JG/pvt	GNM	Unmarried/hostel	Christian/Jacobite
38	Susan	23	JG/pvt	GNM	Unmarried/hostel	Christian/RC
39	Shaiba	30	JG/pvt	GNM	Married/rented	Christian/RC
40	Suja Joseph	26	JG/pvt	GNM	Unmarried/rented	Christian/Jacobite
41	Reena Chacko	26	JG/pvt	GNM	Rented	Christian/Jacobite

42	Ramya Vijayan	26	JG/pvt	Engaged/hostel	Hindu/Ezhava
43	Mini Mathai	24	JG/pvt	Unmarried/hostel	Christian/Pent Christian/Marthoma
44	Sona Mariam	26	JG/pvt	Unmarried/rented	
45	Roja Jacob	27	JG/pvt	Unmarried/rented	Christian/RC
46	Suma Jacob	27	BSA/govt	Unmarried/hostel	Christian/Malankara
47	Navya	27	BSA/govt	Married/quarter	Hindu/Ezhava
48	Sumi	26	BSA/govt	Unmarried/quarter	Hindu/Ezhava
49	Sunila	25	BSA/govt	Unmarried/quarter	Hindu/Ezhava
50	Susanna Kosy	44	BSA/govt	Married/own house	Christian/Jahova's Witnesses
51	Asha	27	BSA/govt	Married/rented	Hindu/Nair
52	Sumitha	27	BSA/govt	Unmarried/quarter with sister and mother	Hindu/Viswakarma
53	Sindhu Madhukumar	34	BSA/govt	Married/quarter	Hindu/Nair

(Continued)

Appendix (*Continued*)

S. No.	Name	Age	Workplace/Names of hospitals	Educational qualification	Marital status/Accommodation	Religion/Caste
54	Rinsy Joy	29	BSA/govt	GNM	Married/rented	Christian/RC
55	Anilakumari	27	BSA/govt	GNM	Married/quarter	Hindu/Nair
56	Anu Jose	30	BSA/govt	GNM	Married/quarter	Christian/RC
57	Soumya	29	BSA/govt	GNM	Unmarried/quarter	Hindu/Nair
58	Grace Cyril	30	BSA/govt	GNM	Married/quarter	Christian/RC
59	Sumangala Devi	36	BSA/govt	GNM	Married/quarter	Hindu/Nair
60	Sony Kurien	30	BSA/govt	GNM	Married/quarter	Christian/RC
61	Annamma Vijayan	47	RML/govt	GNM	Married/quarter	Christian/RC
62	Anitha Varadan	35	RML/govt	GNM	Married/own house	Hindu/Ezhava
63	Ancy Biju	43	RML/govt	GNM	Married/husband's quarter	Christian/RC
64	Anandi	32	RML/govt	GNM	Married/own house	Hindu/Ezhava
65	Liji John	23	AIH/pvt	GNM	Unmarried/hostel	Christian/RC
66	Seena Kurien	24	AIH/pvt	GNM	Unmarried/hostel	Christian/RC
67	Reema Kunjacko	25	AIH/pvt	GNM	Unmarried/hostel	Christian/RC
68	Ruchi	25	AIH/pvt	GNM	Unmarried/hostel	Christian/RC

69	Smriti	23	AIH/pvt	GNM	Unmarried/hostel	Christian/RC
70	Lisa	24	AIH/pvt	GNM	Unmarried/hostel	Christian/RC
71	Molly Padickal	25	AIH/pvt	GNM	Unmarried/hostel	Christian/RC
72	Sushama	24	AIH/pvt	GNM	Unmarried/hostel	Christian/RC
73	Sara Poulose	24	AIH/pvt	GNM	Unmarried/hostel	Christian/RC
74	Lincy Chandi	23	AIH/pvt	GNM	Unmarried/hostel	Christian/RC
75	Teena Philip	25	AIH/pvt	GNM	Unmarried/hostel	Christian/RC
76	Shylaja Aloysius	27	AIH/pvt	GNM	Unmarried/hostel	Christian/LC
77	Jalaja	32	SLJ/pvt	GNM-Kerala-no certificate	Married/rented	Ezhava/Pent
78	Sudha	34	SLJ/pvt	GNM	Married/rented	Hindu/Ezhava
79	Ranjini	23	VNH/pvt	GNM	Unmarried/with cousin	Hindu/Vaniya Vaisyar
80	Parvathy	36	VNH/pvt	GNM	Married to a lab technician/own house	Hindu/Ezhava
81	Sujatha	44	VNH/pvt	GNM	Married/own house	Hindu/Ezhava

(Continued)

Appendix (*Continued*)

S. No.	Name	Age	Workplace/Names of hospitals	Educational qualification	Marital status/Accommodation	Religion/Caste
82	Subha	32	SDCH/pvt	ANM-no certificate	Married/rented	Hindu/ Vaniyavaisyar
83	Shanti	30	SDCH/pvt	ANM	Married/rented	Christian/RC
84	Lallymol	25	VL/pvt	Lab tech course and training and no nursing certificate	Unmarried/with sister	Christian/LC-Pent
85	Lucksy Job	26	VL/pvt	ANM	Unmarried/pvt hostel	Christian/RC
86	Revathi Kuttappan	25	MA/pvt	GNM	Unmarried/hostel	Christian/RC
87	Meera Cherian	26	MA/pvt	GNM	Unmarried/hostel	Christian/RC
88	Nisha	26	MA/pvt	GNM	Unmarried/hostel	Christian/RC
89	Sheeja	27	MA/pvt	GNM	Unmarried/hostel	Christian/RC
90	Neelu George	28	MA/pvt	GNM	Unmarried/hostel	Christian/RC
91	Anna	25	MA/pvt	GNM	Unmarried/hostel	Christian/RC
92	Sanjitha	26	MA/pvt	GNM	Unmarried/hostel	Christian/RC
93	Shaima	25	MA/pvt	GNM	Unmarried/hostel	Christian/RC

94	Sabina	27	MA/pvt	GNM	Unmarried/hostel	Christian/LC
95	Sophia	26	MA/pvt	GNM	Unmarried/hostel	Christian/RC
96	Dolly	27	MA/pvt	GNM	Unmarried/hostel	Christian/RC
97	Shobhana	25	MA/pvt	GNM	Unmarried/hostel	Christian/RC
98	Janani	26	MA/pvt	GNM	Unmarried/hostel	Christian/RC
99	Ananya	23	MA/pvt	GNM	Unmarried/hostel	Christian/RC
100	Mala	24	MA/pvt	GNM	Unmarried/Hostel	Christian/RC
101	Smitha	27	MA/pvt	GNM	Unmarried/hostel	Christian/RC
102	Dhanya	26	HF/pvt	GNM	Unmarried/hostel	Christian/RC
103	Kochurani Joseph	25	HF/pvt	GNM	Unmarried/hostel	Christian/RC
104	Sonia Roy	26	HF/pvt	GNM	Unmarried/hostel	Christian/RC
105	Tiju Varkey	34	HF/pvt	GNM	Married/rented	Christian/RC
106	Jaya Sreekumar	33	HF/pvt	GNM	Married/own house	Hindu/Pillai
107	Binitha	25	MCD/pvt	GNM	Unmarried/rented with cousin	Christian/RC
108	Sajini	23	MCD/pvt	GNM	Unmarried/rented	Christian/Jacobite

(Continued)

Appendix (*Continued*)

S. No.	Name	Age	Workplace/Names of hospitals	Educational qualification	Marital status/Accommodation	Religion/Caste
109	Twinkle Philip	24	MCD/pvt	GNM	Unmarried/rented	Christian/RC
110	Ajitha Mathew	30	MCD/pvt	GNM	**Married/rented**	Christian/RC
111	Ambili	26	MCD/pvt	GNM	Unmarried/rented	Christian/RC
112	Lubina Santoz	25	HA/pvt	GNM	Unmarried/Pvt hostel	Christian/LC
113	Sasmitha	26	HA/pvt	GNM	Unmarried/Pvt hostel	Christian/RC
114	Sanya	26	HA/pvt	ANM	Unmarried/Pvt hostel	Christian/RC
115	Jasmine	29	HA/pvt	GNM	Unmarried/Pvt hostel	Christian/RC
116	Roma	26	HA/pvt	GNM	Unmarried/Pvt hostel	Christian/RC
117	Preethy Paul	25	HA/pvt	GNM	Unmarried/Pvt hostel	Christian/RC
118	Sanila	27	HA/pvt	GNM	Unmarried/rented with sister+Nidhi	Christian/RC
119	Nidhi	25	HA/pvt	GNM	Unmarried/rented	Christian/RC
120	Premalatha	38	SgH/govt	GNM	Married/quarter	Hindu/Nair
121	Rajani	31	SgH/govt	GNM	Married/quarter	Christian/RC

	Name	Age	Hospital	Qualification	Marital/Housing	Religion/Caste
122	Clara Thomas	40	AIIMS/govt	GNM+spl.	Married/quarter	Christian/RC
123	Vanitha Yadav	34	AIIMS/govt	GNM	Married/own house	Christian/RC married to Yadav
124	Helen Xavier	36	AIIMS/govt	GNM	Married/quarter	Christian/RC
125	Tissa Joseph	37	AIIMS/govt	GNM	Married/own house	Christian/RC
126	Suni Saimon	24	Batra/pvt	GNM	Unmarried/hostel	Christian/RC
127	Tushara	27	Batra/pvt	GNM+Spln in OT.	Unmarried/Hostel	Christian/RC
128	Kavitha	28	Batra/pvt	GNM	Unmarried/rented	Christian/RC
129	Priya Lasar	26	Batra/pvt	GNM	Unmarried/hostel	Christian/LC
130	Lovely	25	JNH/pvt	GNM	Unmarried/rented	Christian/RC
131	Veena	26	JNH/pvt	GNM	Unmarried/rented with cousin	Hindu/Ezhava
132	Supriya	27	SNH/pvt	GNM	Unmarried/rented with cousin	Hindu/Ezhava
133	Lavanya Maxim	26	Max/pvt	GNM	Unmarried/hostel	Christian/LC

(Continued)

Appendix (*Continued*)

S. No.	Name	Age	Workplace/Names of hospitals	Educational qualification	Marital status/Accommodation	Religion/Caste
134	Chintha Balan	26	Max/pvt	GNM	Unmarried/hostel	Hindu/Ezhava
135	Rasmi Oscar	26	Max/pvt	GNM	Unmarried/hostel	Christian/LC
136	Pushpa Suresh	30	FH/pvt	ANM training/no certificate	Married/own house	Hindu/Vaniya Vaisyar
137	Kavya	28	FH/pvt	No training/getting trained	Unmarried/hostel	Christian/RC
138	Latha	31	FH/pvt	ANM	Married/hostel	Christian/RC
139	Suchitra	27	FH/pvt	ANM	Unmarried/hostel	Hindu/Nair
140	Usha	28	FH/pvt	ANM	Unmarried/hostel	Hindu/Ezhava
141	Amala Soman	27	RGCC/pvt	GNM	Unmarried/with cousin/BSA	Hindu/Ezhava
142	Simi	25	RGCC/pvt	GNM	Unmarried/hostel	Christian/RC
143	Pratibha	24	RGCC/pvt	GNM	Unmarried/hostel	Christian/RC
144	Manjusha	25	RGCC/pvt	GNM	Unmarried/hostel	Hindu/Ezhava
145	Fabina	24	RGCC/pvt	GNM	Unmarried/hostel	Christian/RC

146	Swapna	27	RGCC/pvt	GNM	Unmarried/rented	Christian/RC
147	Sinimol	26	RGCC/pvt	GNM	Unmarried/rented	Christian/RC
148	Prabha Joshy Parayil	25	RGCC/pvt	GNM	Unmarried/rented	Christian/RC
149	Sandhya Joseph	26	RGCC/pvt	GNM	Unmarried/rented	Christian/RC
150	Kochumol V. Jose	27	RGCC/pvt	GNM	Unmarried/hostel	Christian/RC

* Names changed to keep the anonymity but bear a resemblance to the original name that in many cases reflect religious identity or community practice of naming people

** SGR-Sri Ganga Ram; SM-Shanti Mukand; JG-Jaipur Golden; BSA-Baba Sahib Ambedkar; RML-Ram Manohar Lohia; AIH-Apollo Indraprastha Hospital; VNH-Vinayaka Nursing Home; SDCH-Sanathana Dharma Charitable Hospital; VL-Vasant Lok; MA-Maharaja Agrasen; SLJ-Sunderlal Jain; HF-Holy Family; MCD-Mata Chanan Devi; HA-Holy Angels; SgH- Safdarjung Hospital; AIIMS-All India Institute of Medical Sciences; JNS-Jeevan Nursing Home; SNH-Shakti Nursing Home; FH-Family Hospital: RGCC-Rajiv Gandhi Cancer Centre : pvt-Private sector; govt-Public sector

*** GNM-General Nursing and Midwifery; ANM-Auxiliary Nursing and Midwifery; spl-Specialisation

**** Chr-Christian; RC-Roman Catholic; Orth-Orthodox; Pent.-Pentecostal; LC-Latin Catholic

Bibliography

Abbott, A. 1988. *The System of Professions: An Essay on the Division of Expert Labor.* Chicago: Chicago Press.

Abraham, M. 1996. *Religion, Caste and Gender: Missionaries and Nursing History in South India.* Madras: B.I. Publications.

Agrawal, A. 2006. 'Introduction: Women, Work and Migration in Asia', in Anuja Agrawal (ed.), *Migrant Women and Work.* New Delhi: Sage Publications.

Anderson, B. 1983. *Imagined Communities: Reflections on the Origin and Spread of Nationalism.* London: Verso.

Aravamudan, G. 1975. 'Nurses and Nuns from Kerala', in D. Jain (ed.), *Indian Women*, pp. 263–70. New Delhi: Ministry of Information and Broadcasting.

Baly, M.E. 1987. 'The Nightingale Nurses: The Myth and the Reality', in C. Maggs (ed.), *Nursing History The state of the Art*, pp. 33–59. London: Croom Helm.

Barber, P.G. 2000. 'Agency in Philippine Women's Migration and Provisional Diaspora', *Women's Studies International Forum* (Special Issue: *Gender Politics and Diasporic Identities of the Asia-Pacific*), 23(4): 399–411.

Baru, R. 2004. 'Privatisation of Healthcare: Conditions of Workers in Private Hospitals', in M. Bhattacharya (ed.), *Globalisation,* pp. 81–86. New Delhi:Tulika.

———. 2005. 'Gender and Social Characteristics of the Labour Force in Health Services', in S. Kak and B. Pati (eds), *Exploring Gender Equations Colonial and Post Colonial India*, pp. 281–99. New Delhi: Nehru Memorial Museum and Library.

Bernstein B. 1971. 'On the Classification and Framing of Educational Knowledge', in M.F.D. Young (ed.), *Knowledge and Control: New Directions for the Sociology of Education*, pp. 47–69. London: Collier-Macmillan.

Bourdieu, P. 1977. *Outline of a Theory of Practice.* Cambridge & New York: Cambridge University Press.

Bullough, V.L. and B. Bullough. 1978. *Care of the Sick: The Emergence of Modern Nursing.* London: Croom Helm.

Burawoy, M. 2000. 'Introduction', in M. Burawoy (ed.), *Global Ethnography:Forces, Connections, and Imaginations in a Post-modern World*, pp. 1–35. Berkeley: University of California Press.

Carter, R. and G. Kirkup. 1990. *Women in Engineering: A Good Place to Be.* London: Macmillan.

Chanana, K. 2001. *Interrogating Women's Education: Bounded Visions, Expanding Horizons.* New Delhi: Rawat Publications.

Chatterjee, P. 1994a. 'Whose Imagined Community?' in P. Chatterjee (ed.), *Nation and its Fragments*, pp. 3–13. New Delhi: Oxford University Press.

———. 1994b. 'Nation and Its Women', in P. Chatterjee (ed.), *Nation and its Fragments*, pp. 116–34. New Delhi: Oxford University Press.

Deere, C.D. and M. León de Leal. 1981. 'Peasant Production, Proletarianization, and the Sexual Division of Labor in the Andes', *SIGNS: Journal of Women in Culture and Society*, 7 (2): 338–60.

Devika, J. 2005. 'The Malayali Sexual Revolution: Sex, 'Liberation' and Family Planning in Kerala', *Contributions to Indian Sociology*, 39(3): 343–74.

———. 2007. *En-Gendering Individuals The Language of Re-forming in Twentieth Century Keralam.* New Delhi: Orient Longman.

Devine, P. 1989. 'Stereotypes and Prejudice: Their Automatic and Controlled Components', *Journal of Personality and Social Psychology*, 56: 5–18.

Dhaulta, J.P. 2001. 'The Trained Nurses' Association of India' in Trained Nurses Association of India (ed.), *History and Trends in Nursing in India*, pp. 210–26. New Delhi: TNAI.

Eapen, M. and P. Kodoth. 2003. 'Family Structure, Women's Education and Work: Re-Examining the High Status of Women in Kerala', in S. Mukhopadhyay and R. Sudarshan (eds), *Tracking Gender Equity under Economic Reforms*, pp. 227–68. New Delhi: Kali for Women.

Fitzgerald, R. 1997. 'Rescue and Redemption: The Rise of Female Medical Missions in Colonial India during the Late Nineteenth and Early Twentieth Century', in A. M. Rafferty (ed.), *Nursing History and the Politics of Welfare*, pp. 64–79. London: Routledge.

Forbes, G. 1981. 'The Indian Women's Movement: A Struggle for Women's Rights or National Liberation?' in G. Minault (ed.), *The Extended family Women and Political Participation in India and Pakistan*, pp. 49–82. Delhi: Chanakya Publications.

———. 1996. *Women in Modern India.* New Delhi: Foundation Books.

———. 2005a. 'Managing Midwifery in India', in G. Forbes (ed.), *Women in Colonial India*, pp. 79–100. New Delhi: Chronicle Books.

Fruzzetti, L. 2006. 'Kinship Issues and Issues of Nationalism Issues of Female Abandonment in Calcutta', in L. Fruzzetti and S. Tenhunen (eds), *Culture, Power and Agency: Gender in Indian Ethnography*, pp. 1–20. Kolkata: Stree.

Fruzzetti, L. and S. Tenhunen. 2006. 'Introduction', in L. Fruzzetti and S. Tenhunen (eds), *Culture, Power and Agency: Gender in Indian Ethnography*, pp. vii–xxiii. Kolkata: Stree.

Gallo, E. 2008. 'Unorthodox Sisters: Gender Relations and Generational Change among Malayali Migrants in Italy', in R. Palriwala and P. Uberoi (eds), *Marriage, Migration, and Gender*. New Delhi: Sage Publications.

Georges, E. 1992. 'Women's Experiences in a Transnational Community: Gender, Class and Migration in the Dominican Republic', in *Annals of the New York*, Academy of Sciences.

George, S. 2000. '"Dirty Nurses" and 'Men who Play'', in M. Burawoy (ed.), *Global Ethnography: Forces, Connections, and Imaginations in a Postmodern World*, pp. 144–74. Berkeley: University of California Press.

———. 2005. *When Women Come First Gender and Class in Transnational Migration*. Berkeley: University of California Press.

Ghosh, J. 2004. 'The Changing Nature of Women's Work under Globalisation: A Consideration of Recent Trends in Asia', *The Voice of the Working Woman*, 24(12): 17–19.

Goldbart, J. and D. Hustler. 2005. 'Ethnography', in B. Somekh and C. Lewin (eds), *Research Methods in the Social Sciences: A Guide for Students and Researchers*, pp.16–21. London: Sage Publications.

Gregor, F.M. 1994. 'Nurses' Educative Work: Constructing the Medical Hierarchy', in B.S. Bolaria and R. Bolaria (eds), *Women, Medicine and Health*, pp. 219–30. Halifax: Fernwood Publishing.

Grusky, D.B. (ed.). 1994. *Social Stratification: Class, Race and Gender in Sociological Perspectives*. Oxford: Westview Press.

Gulani, K.K. 2001. 'Development of Nursing Education in India', in Trained Nurses Association of India (ed.), *History and Trends in Nursing in India*, pp. 140–73. New Delhi: TNAI.

Gulati, L. 1993. *In the Absence of their Men: The Impact of Male Migration on Women*. New Delhi: Sage Publications.

Gulati, L. 1997. 'Social Consequences of Male Migration Case Studies of Women Left behind', in K.C. Zachariah and S.I. Rajan (eds), *Kerala's Demographic Transition Determinants and Consequences*. New Delhi: Sage Publications.

Harding, S. 1993. 'Rethinking Standpoint Epistemology What is 'Strong Objectivity?'', in L. Alcoff and E. Potter (eds), *Feminist Epistemologies*, pp. 49–82. New York: Routledge.

Harzig, C. 2001. 'Women Migrants as Global and Local Agents', in P. Sharpe (ed.), *Women, Gender and Labour Migration: Historical and Global Perspectives*, pp. 15–28. London: Routledge.

Hawker, R. 1987. 'For the Good of the Patient?', in C. Maggs (ed.), *Nursing History The state of the Art*, pp. 143–52. London: Croom Helm.

Healey, M. Unpublished. 'Nursing in Independent India: An Examination of Exclusion', Australia: La Trobe University.

Hoffman, C. and N. Hurst (1990). 'Gender Stereotypes: Perception or Rationalization?' *Journal of Personality and Social Psychology*, 58: 197–208.

Jaiswal, R.P. 1988. 'Women in Science and Engineering Professions in India: A Case Study of Unequal Participation', Workshop 2–5 November, Indian Institute of Sciences, Bangalore.

Jeffrey, R. 1992. *Politics, Women and Well-being: How Kerala Became "a Model"*. London: Macmillan.

John, M.E. 2008. 'Gender Gaps' in Higher Education: A Note on Recent Data' in *Anchoring Women's Studies in India*, 25 years of The Indian Association for Women's Studies, A Commemoration, pp. 55–63. Delhi: IAWS.

Kabir, M. 2003. 'Beyond Philanthropy: The Rockefeller Foundation's Public Health Intervention in Thiruvithamkoor, 1929–1939', Working Paper 350, Thiruvananthapuram: CDS.

Kabeer, N. 2007. 'Marriage, Motherhood and Masculinity in the Global Economy: The Emerging Crisis in Social Reproduction', J.P. Naik Memorial Lecture, CWDS, New Delhi.

Kaufman, D.R. 1984. 'Professional Women: How Real are the Recent Gains?', in J. Freeman (ed.), *Women A Feminist Perspective*. California: Mayfield.

Keller, E.F. 1995. *Gender and Science: Origin, History and Politics*, reprint, Osiris No. 10, pp. 27–38.

Kellner, D. and J. Share. 2005. 'Toward Critical Media Literacy: Core Concepts, Debates, Organizations, and Policy', *Discourse: Studies in the Cultural Politics of Education*, 26(3): 369–86.

Kergoat, D., F. Imbert, H. L. Doaré and D. Senotier (eds). 1992. *Les Infirmieres et Leur Coordination 1988–1989*. Paris: Lamarre.

Khadria, B. 2006. 'International Recruitment of Nurses in India: Implications of Stakeholder Perspectives on Overseas Labour Markets, Migration, and Return', Working Paper No. 68, Asia Research Institute, Singapore.

Kodoth, P. 2007. 'Rendering Livelihoods Insecure: Dowry and Female Seclusion in Left Developmental Contexts, West Bengal and Kerala', in M. Krishnaraj (ed.), *Gender, Food Security and Rural Livelihoods*. Calcutta: Stree.

Krishnaraj, M. 1991. *Women and Science: Selected Essay*. Mumbai: Himalaya Publishing House.

Kukreja, S. 1995. 'The Political Economy of the Feminisation of the Tertiary in Developing Countries: Some Cross-national Findings', in M.S. Das and V.K. Gupta (eds), *Social Status of Women in Developing Countries*, pp. 15–34. New Delhi: MD Publications.

Kurien, J. 1995. 'The Kerala Model: Its Central Tendency and the Outlier', *Social Scientist*, 23(1–3): 70–90.

Kurup, S. 2006. 'Four Women India Forgot', *The Times of India*, 7 May.

Lazarus, H. 1945. 'The All India Women's Conference Tract No. 5', Our Nursing Services, Aundh.

Lindberg, A. 2001. *Experience and Identity: A Historical Account of Class, Caste, and Gender among the Cashew Workers of Kerala, 1930–2000*. Lund: Department of History at Lund University.

Madan T.N., P. Wiebe, R. Said, and M. Dias. 1980. *Doctors and Society: Asian Case Studies India, Malaysia, Sri Lanka*. New Delhi: Vikas.

Maggs, C. 1987. *Nursing History: The State of the Art*. London: Croom Helm.

Malhotra, A. 2003. 'Of Dais and Midwives: 'Middle-class' Interventions in the Management of Women's Reproductive Health—A Study from Colonial Punjab', *Indian Journal of Gender Studies*, 10(2): 229–59.

Marks, S. 1994. *Divided Sisterhood Race, Class and Gender in the South African Nursing Profession*. Johannesburg: Witwatersrand University Press.

Mayoux, L. 2001. 'Tackling the Downside: Social Capital, Women's Empowerment and Micro-finance in Cameroon', *Development and Change*, 32(3): 435–64.

Mazumdar, V. 1990. 'The Social Reform Movement in India-From Ranade to Nehru', in B.R. Nanda (ed.), *Indian Women From Purdah to Modernity*, pp. 41–66. Delhi: Radiant Publishers.

Menon, N. 1992. 'Women in Trade Unions: A Study of AITUC, INTUC and CITU in the Seventies', in S. Gothoskar (ed.), *Struggle of Women at Work*, pp. 187–96. New Delhi: Vikas.

Milkman, R. (ed.). 1985. *Women, Work and Protest: A Century of U.S. Women's Labor History*. Boston: Routledge and Kegan Paul.

Minocha, A. 1996. *Perceptions and Interactions in a Medical Setting: A Sociological Study of Women's Hospital*. New Delhi: Hindustan Publishers.

Mohan, S.N. 1985. *Status of Nurses in India*. New Delhi: Uppal.

Morrison, B.M. 1997. 'The Embourgeoisement of the Kerala Farmer', *Modern Asian Studies*, 31(1): 61–87.

Mukhopadhyay, C.C. 1994. 'Family Structure and Indian Women's Participation in Science and Engineering', in C.C. Mukhopadhyay and S. Seymour (eds) pp. 103–32 in *Women, Education and Family Structure in India*. Boulder: Westview Press.

Mukhopadhyay, C.C. and S. Seymour. 1994. 'Introduction and Theoretical Overview', in C.C. Mukhopadhyay and S. Seymour (ed.), *Women, Education and Family Structure in India*, pp. 1–34. Boulder: Westview Press.

Mukhopadhyay, S. 2007. 'Understanding the Enigma of Women's Status in Kerala: Does High Literacy Necessarily Translate into High Status?' in S. Mukhopadhyay (ed.), *The Enigma of the Kerala Women: A Failed Promise of Literacy*, pp. 3–31. New Delhi: Social Science Press.

Mukhopadhyay S., J. Basu and S.I. Rajan. 2007. 'Mental Health, Gender Ideology and Women's Status in Kerala', in S. Mukhopadhyay (ed.), *The Enigma of the Kerala Women: A Failed Promise of Literacy*, pp. 71–101. New Delhi: Social Science Press.

Nagpal, N. 2001a. 'Establishment of Significant Hospitals and Nursing Training Schools (1664–1947)', in Trained Nurses Association of India (ed.), *History and Trends in Nursing in India*, pp. 22–58. New Delhi: TNAI.

———. 2001b. 'Development of Nursing and Healthcare 1947–2000', in Trained Nurses Association of India (ed.), *History and Trends in Nursing in India*, pp. 59–139. New Delhi: TNAI.

Nair, S. 1998. 'Social Context of Girls' Schooling in Kerala a Study of Malabar Region 1900–1950', MPhil Dissertation, Jawaharlal Nehru University, New Delhi.

———. 2004. 'Gender, Education and Work: A Study of Women Engineers in Kerala'. PhD Dissertation, Jawaharlal Nehru University, New Delhi.

———. 2007. 'Rethinking Citizenship, Community and Rights: The Case of Nurses from Kerala in Delhi', *Indian Journal of Gender Studies*, 14(1): 137–56.

———. 2010. 'Nurses' Strikes in Delhi: A Status Question', *Economic and Political Weekly*, xlv(14): 23–25.

Nair, S. and M. Healey. 2006. 'A Profession on the Margins: Status Issues in Indian Nursing', Occasional Paper No.45, CWDS, New Delhi.

Nair, S. and M. Percot. 2007. 'Transcending Boundaries: Indian Nurses in Internal and International Migration', Occasional Paper No. 47, CWDS. New Delhi.

Namboodiripad, E.M.S. 1984. *Political Realignment in Kerala Society and Politics: An Historical Survey*. New Delhi: National Book Centre.

Nelson, J.A. 1996. *Feminism, Objectivity and Economics.* London: Routledge.

Oommen, M.A. 1999. 'Introduction', in M.A. Oommen (ed.), *Rethinking Development Kerala's Development Experience*, vol. 1. New Delhi: Concept.

Oommen, T.K. 1978. *Doctors and Nurses A Study in Occupational Role Structure.* Delhi: Macmillan.

Osella, F. and C. Osella. 2000. Migration, Money and Masculinity in Kerala, *The Journal of the Royal Anthropological Institute*, 6(1): 117–133.

Osella C. and Osella F. 2006. *Men and Masculinities in South India.* London: Anthem Press.

Parikh P.P. and S.P. Sukhatme. 1992. *Women Engineers in India.* Bombay: Indian Institute of Technology.

Pedraza, S. 1991. 'Women and Migration: The Social Consequences of Gender', *Annual Review of Sociology*, 17: 303–25.

Percot, M. 2005. 'Les infirmières indiennes émigrées dans le Golfe: de l'opportunité à la stratégie', *Revue Européenne des Migrations Internationales,* 21(1): 29–54.

———. 2006. 'From Opportunity to Life strategy: Indian Nurses in the Gulf', in A. Agrawal (ed.), *Migrant Women and Work*, pp. 155–76. New Delhi: Sage Publications.

Pringle, R. 1998. *Sex and Medicine: Gender, Power, and Authority in the Medical Profession.* Cambridge: Cambridge University Press.

Raghavachari, R. 1990. *Conflicts and Adjustments: Indian Nurses in an Urban Milieu.* Delhi: Academic Foundation.

Raju, S. 2007. 'More Unequal than Others: Gender Differentials in Access to Higher Education, State and District Level Patterns', University Grants Commission Report, New Delhi.

Roy, M. 2005. 'Ants in the Pants' in S. Basu (ed.), *Dowry and Inheritance.* New Delhi: Women Unlimited.

Saradamoni, K. 1995. 'Crisis in the Fishing Industry and Women's Migration: The Case of Kerala', in L. Schenk-Sandbergen (ed.), *Women and Seasonal Migration*, pp. 155–209. New Delhi: Sage Publications.

———. 2005. 'Progressive Land Legislations and Subordination of Women', in S. Basu (ed.), *Dowry and Inheritance*, pp. 214–23. New Delhi: Women Unlimited.

Sarasúa, C. 2001. 'Leaving Home to Help Family? Temporary Migrants in Eighteenth and Nineteenth-Century Spain', in P. Sharpe (ed.), *Gender and Labour Migration: Historical and Global Perspectives*, pp. 29–59. London: Routledge.

Senotier, D. 1992. 'Cent ans d'évolution de la profession', in Kergoat, D. et al. (eds), *Les Infirmieres et Leur Coordination 1988–1989*. Paris : Lamarre.

Sharpe, P. 2001. 'Introduction: Gender and the Experience of Migration', in P.Sharpe (ed.), *Women, Gender and Labour Migration: Historical and Global Perspectives*, pp. 1–14. London: Routledge.

Silvey, R. and R. Elmhirst. 2003. 'Engendering Social Capital: Women Workers and Rural-Urban Networks in Indonesia's Crisis', *World Development*, 31(5): 865–81.

Skeldon, R. 2003. 'Interlinkages between Internal and International Migration and Development in National Migration and Development', Economic and Social Commission for Group Meeting on Migration and Development, 27–29 August, Bangkok.

Smith, D.E. 1989. 'Writing Patriarchy', in R.A. Wallace (ed.), *Feminism and Sociological Theory*, pp. 34–64. New Delhi: Sage Publications.

———. 2007. 'Institutional Ethnography', in S.N. Hesse-Biber (ed.), *Institutional Ethnography Theory and Praxis*, pp. 409–16. New Delhi: Sage Publications.

Special Correspondent. 2005. 'Do Not Impose Biased Criteria for Nursing Admission', Many institutions denying admission to married women November 25. *The Hindu*.

Subrahmanyan, L. 1998. *Women Scientists in the Third World The Indian Experience*. New Delhi: Sage Publications.

Tamale, S. 1999. *When Hens Begin To Crow: Gender and Parliamentary Politics In Uganda*. Boulder: Westview Press.

Thapan, M. 2005. 'Series Introduction', in M. Thapan (ed.), *Transnational Migration and the Politics of Identity*, pp. 9–20. New Delhi: Sage Publications.

Tharakan, P.K. 1984. 'Socio-economic Factors in Educational Development Case of 19th Century Travancore', *Economic and Political Weekly*, xix(45): 1913–28; xix(46): pp.1959–67.

Times News Network. 2007. 'Hospitals are Sick, Asserts CAG Report; 'Lagging in Many Areas', *The Times of India*, April 21, Delhi.

Timmons, S. and L. East. 2011. 'Uniforms, Status and Professional Boundaries in Hospital', *Sociology of Health and Illness*, 33(7): 1035–1049.

Trained Nurses Association of India (TNAI). 2000. *Handbook of the TNAI*. New Delhi: TNAI.

Viswanath, K. and S. Tandon-Mehrotra. 2007. 'Shall We Go Out?' Women's Safety in Public Spaces in Delhi', *Economic and Political Weekly*, 42(17): 1542–48.

Weber, M. 1994. 'Status Groups and Classes', in D.B. Grusky (ed.), *Social Stratification: Class, Race and Gender in Sociological Perspectives,* pp. 122–26. Oxford: Westview Press.

Wilkinson, A. 2001. 'Military Nursing', in Trained Nurses Association of India (ed.), *History and Trends in Nursing in India,* pp. 8–21. New Delhi: TNAI.

Witz, A. 1992. *Professions and Patriarchy.* London: Routledge.

Workers Solidarity. 2000. *Critical Condition: A Report on Workers in Delhi's Private Hospitals,* Workers Solidarity, New Delhi.

Zachariah, K.C., E.T. Mathew and S.I. Rajan. 2003. *Dynamics of Migration in Kerala: Dimensions, Differentials and Consequences.* Hyderabad: Orient Longman.

Zachariah, K.C and S.I. Rajan. 2004. 'Gulf Revisited Economic Consequences of Emigration from Kerala Emigration and Unemployment'. Working Paper 363, Thiruvananthapuram: Centre for Development Studies.

Online Resources

Boyd, M. and E. Grieco. 2003. 'Women and Migration: Incorporating Gender into International Migration Theory', http://www.migration information.org/Feature/print.cfm?ID=106.

'Shanti Mukand case Judgement opens a can of Worms', http://www. expresshealthcaremgmt.com/200701/market13.shtml (last accessed on 18 September 2008).

Wajihuddin, M. 2006. 'When Nurses are Muslims', http://articles. timesofindia.indiatimes.com/2006-12-17/india/27813741_1_ nursing-school-muslim-girls-profession.

http://www.delhigovt.nic.in/dept/health/hospital.asp (last accessed on 11 April 2005).

http://www.cscsarchive.org/MediaArchive/medialaw.nsf/1105 fec5535ec8ab6525698d00258968/1c65a18ee3460a4d6525729c 0025222b/$FILE/A0160155.pdf (last accessed on 11 December 2008).

About the Author

Sreelekha Nair is Junior Fellow at the Centre for Women's Development Studies, New Delhi. Prior to this, she was Research Associate at the Centre. She completed her PhD from Jawaharlal Nehru University, New Delhi. She was awarded the Hermes Post-Doctoral fellowship by Fondation maison des sciences de l'homme, Paris to pursue her research at the Centre national de la recherche scientifique. Her research interests include sociology of professions, women and work, migration and data restitution in women's studies.

Index

9 781138 662582